THE IMAGINARY PATIENT

Jules Montague

The Imaginary Patient

How Diagnosis Gets Us Wrong

GRANTA

Granta Publications, 12 Addison Avenue, London W11 4QR

First published in Great Britain by Granta Books, 2022

A CIP catalogue record for this book is available from the British Library.

1 3 5 7 9 10 8 6 4 2

ISBN 978 1 78378 584 1 (hardback)
ISBN 978 1 78378 586 5 (ebook)

Typeset by Avon DataSet Ltd, Alcester, Warwickshire B49 6HN
Printed and bound by CPI Group (UK) Ltd, Croydon, CR0 4YY

www.granta.com

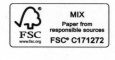

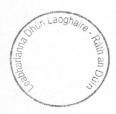

Contents

Prologue

I meet Joyce during one of my ward rounds at a hospital in Beira, Mozambique. I work in this port town, where the Pungwe river meets the Indian Ocean, for a month each year. Most nights are marked by the buzz of mosquitoes and the scuttling of cockroaches in my guesthouse by Ponta Gea. Early each morning as I walk to the hospital, I see fishermen by Macúti beach lighthouse, casting their nets into the gleaming waters. Drivers in their green and yellow *tchopelas* (autorickshaws), horns blaring and music reverberating, speed down streets marked by faded colonial grandeur. Traders make their way to hawk fruit and vegetables at Mercado do Goto.

A year from now, in 2019, Cyclone Idai will make landfall here, followed six weeks later by Cyclone Kenneth, killing at least 600 people across the country and destroying at least 70% of Beira's buildings.

Joyce is in her sixties, and wearied by a long battle with tuberculosis that has marked these later years of hers. She has beaten the odds already in some ways – life expectancy is less than fifty in Beira – yet now a new set of symptoms has brought her back to this medical ward. Pain contorts her body, dizziness brings her to her knees, weakness has left her limbs almost useless. But blood test results and X-rays are unremarkable; there is no evidence of an infection or inflammation or anything else to explain her ill health. As Joyce sleeps that afternoon, her husband tells us that a healer in their ancestral home in central Mozambique has already identified the cause of her sickness. He has decreed that Joyce is possessed by a spirit. One of the local hospital doctors, Ricardo, tells me how these spirits have declared themselves in the bodies of women like Joyce.

Mozambique gained independence from Portugal in 1975 after more than a decade of armed struggle, but the newly liberated nation was fractured and fragile. During a civil war between 1977 and 1992 that saw one million deaths, Joyce was subjected to forced labour at a time when rape and sexual slavery were common as weapons of war. In the aftermath of that war, the *gamba* – the spirits of murdered young soldiers – returned to earth to seek justice. They searched for those who killed them or their families, or those who consumed medications made from their corpses (based on a belief that these medications would confer protection from violence).

Ricardo had seen several patients like this – women who underwent severe trauma and much later developed somatic symptoms. Joyce's husband held out hope for a cure. He had asked the village's *gamba* healer to conduct a ceremony in the coming days. The healer would draw the spirit from Joyce's body towards him, and re-enact the experiences of the soldier: crawling and running, fighting and fainting. Then the spirit would return to Joyce, causing her to scream and her body to spasm violently. Next, the healer would appeal to the spirit, appease him, listen to his suffering. The family had to acknowledge their wrongdoings during the war. Only then could the *gamba* depart Joyce's body, only then could her recovery begin.

In the UK, we might diagnose Joyce with post-traumatic stress disorder (PTSD), and say that her symptoms and flashbacks are markers of deep psychological distress in the wake of conflict. But I wonder if this label truly captures her experiences. In fact, the designation of *gamba* possession appears to me to run much deeper than a series of diagnostic PTSD bullet points ever could. It acknowledges the specificities of a brutal and protracted civil war and allows for a ceremony where families can be reconciled and injustices can be addressed. It enables remembering in a society where a convenient collective amnesia has taken hold.

Is one explanation of Joyce's distress more valid than another? Spirit possession has no scientific markers – genetic predisposition or brain-scan findings, for instance – to prove or disprove it as a diagnosis. But neither does PTSD. Are these two labels simply two sides of the same coin? Both relate to a similar set of symptoms in the aftermath of trauma, but at first glance, PTSD undervalues the cultural currency of Joyce's experiences, and her community's too. Most importantly, spirit possession is an explanation that Joyce believes in, it speaks to what she has lived through. In some societies, spirits are seen as wholly vengeful, and possession is stigmatised and punished disproportionately in women, but there is no singular narrative of hostility and vindictiveness around *gamba*. Possession is itself associated with suffering, but the ceremony that awaits Joyce carries the potential for cure. Even if a *gamba* spirit remains within Joyce's body afterwards, she will become a healer herself and then, in contrast to traditional local expectations that a wife is subordinate to her husband, her husband must subordinate himself, via the spirit, to Joyce. He may even be described in the community as '*mwamuna inei ha hana ndzero*' ('a man without ideas'). Typically, though, mutual trust and respect are demanded, and women healers have a kind of protected status. If the occasion demands it, they are encouraged to sing the words other women in the community cannot: '*Djongwe lika penga gwanda mussoroi*' ('when the cock goes crazy, cut off his head'). In Joyce's case, there was one diagnosis, tuberculosis, which remained seemingly irrefutable and universal, but her somatic symptoms were open to interpretation. Her story, when I heard it that day in Beira, made me wonder: what is the point of a diagnosis – the label we give to a disease – if it cannot be reliable over time or valid across space, or if it fails to encompass our culture and beliefs? How could a diagnosis, a construct I had learnt to think of as relatively static and stable, vary so dramatically according to religion, ritual and region?

During my clinical practice, I continued to face the same questions repeatedly. Not just in neurology (my own speciality) or psychiatry (PTSD is a psychiatric diagnosis), but across other medical specialities too. The concept of diagnosis – which is, after all, at the root of medicine, its primary tool – seemed to be deeply flawed. Diagnosis, in my mind, was supposed to bring order to chaos, but I found when I returned to the UK that my faith in its universality and utility floundered, particularly when I thought of Joyce's journey in Beira.

What if the seemingly straightforward diagnoses I made in London – cancer, dementia, schizophrenia, multiple sclerosis – were also not quite as they seemed? What if diagnoses themselves, rather than the treatments for them, were harmful to those I was trying to help? As I began to doubt my hitherto straightforward belief in this quintessential tool of medical practice, I initially searched for answers through my own patients. But I soon realised that I would have to travel further afield – to police stations, prisons, psychiatric hospitals and refugee camps. With each story I unearthed, I was transported back to Joyce in Beira. There, I had begun to question whether a diagnosis of PTSD – a label couched in western terms – would not have considered the context of Joyce's distress. A diagnosis that ignored her belief in spirit possession may even have impeded her recovery, by failing to grant her agency within her community and neglecting the possibility of societal reconciliation and renewal. It could have represented a kind of imposition, perhaps even a form of cultural imperialism.

Instead, she had left hospital that evening with an explanation of her symptoms that she and her family believed in: a healer awaited her, and hopefully recovery too.

Introduction

London, 1817: James Parkinson, an apothecary and general physician, sits in his consulting rooms at 1 Hoxton Square. It's a basement office, so through the window his view of each passer-by is mainly of legs striding and arms swinging and shoulders hunching. A man shuffles by, the top of his spine as curved as a 'carp fishing hook'. Later, a stooped woman walks across the square, her left hand visibly trembling by her side. Over the days and weeks, a pattern seems to form, a constellation of signs, the beginnings of a description.

He stops some of these strangers in the street, a matter of 'casual observation', he later writes. And in them he sees striking similarities: 'extremities that were considerably agitated', 'the body much bowed and shaken', 'the speech [...] very much interrupted'. His *Essay on the Shaking Palsy* tells the stories of six of these patients. Published that year by Sherwood, Neely and Jones of London and printed by Whittingham and Rowland, priced at 3 shillings, in sixty-six pages it gives the first ever comprehensive description of the eponymous disease.

Over 200 years later, I would diagnose Parkinson's through similar observations, albeit in a windowless clinic room in North London rather than looking out on Hoxton Square.

'This 67-year-old, Mrs Adebayo, has been falling frequently,' read the letter of referral from her GP. 'Her walking has slowed up.

Her writing is smaller than it was before.' The GP already had her suspicions. Now I did too. I watched for a characteristic shake of the hand as Mrs Adebayo walked into my clinic room. And there it was – a pill-rolling tremor, we call it. The rhythmic circular motion of the thumb as it makes contact with the index finger. I watched for a stooped and shuffling gait too. I asked about her sense of smell – yes, she hadn't quite been able to smell her morning coffee for the past year. I confirmed she was talking and lashing out in her sleep. The clues were building. When the patterns are consistently visible, we give them diagnostic labels. My ability to apply this one relies on the work done by James Parkinson in Hoxton Square, on the stories he carefully gathered and the patterns he detected.

Almost every consultation plays out in this way. Mr Brophy was ninety-eight years old. Every evening in his Camden flat, he saw an army of silent soldiers marching through his kitchen. A phalanx of St Bernard dogs formed a guard of honour. Mr Brophy knew the soldiers weren't real. Same for the dogs. He remained silent, letting them pass through his home all the same.

I examined Mr Brophy's eyes.

Symptom (the subjective experience perceived only by the patient): seeing things that weren't really there, i.e. visual hallucinations.

Sign (the observable evidence of disease): bilateral cataracts.

Diagnosis: Charles Bonnet syndrome, secondary to visual impairment.

This diagnostic label is shorthand for the nature of the condition and its potential evolution. In Mr Brophy's case, I could reassure him that it was benign and that removing his cataracts might well resolve it.

Mr Brophy reminded me that he was nearly a hundred years old, and said he was perfectly happy to have brave fighters and beautiful St Bernards drop into his flat each evening. His wife had died two years before; they had been married for seventy-five years. The soldiers and the dogs kept him company.

Diagnostic labels are intended to provide a common language between medics, over centuries and across borders. They allow us to communicate with patients, and patients to communicate with one another. They propel research that elucidates pathology – the causes and effects of disease – and onwards the journey goes towards treatment, perhaps even a cure.

However, not all our symptoms lead to a diagnosis. Instead, our personal experience of our symptoms takes us to a doctor. Illness – a personal account – is what we feel and speak of; it is the narrative we impart, shaped by the culture we live in. The doctor may detect a disease – some sort of malfunction in our physical or psychological process, a recognisable pattern, sometimes with measurable consequences, for instance an abnormal blood test or chest X-ray. The label then provided for that disease is a diagnosis. Doctors have pre-existing categories at the ready when a patient presents to them, and so sometimes illnesses become diseases and diseases become diagnoses. When a patient's illness is not labelled with a diagnosis (by a doctor), they might experience a prevailing sense of relief. But sometimes there is a sense of rejection instead – the medical establishment has failed to recognise individual distress, pain, disability; now the patient's family, friends and co-workers may do so too. 'They must think there's nothing wrong with me,' the dismissed patient thinks.

Diagnosis, then, is the tool whereby a person becomes a patient officially embedded in the medical system, eligible for treatment (or at risk of being subjected to it) and worthy of receiving a prognosis – an account of the likely progress or outcome of a condition – if one can be deduced.

Contemporary diagnoses are usually reached by consensus.

Scientists and doctors notice a characteristic clinical picture taking form – a constellation of symptoms and signs. They publish their descriptions of a 'typical patient' in journals and textbooks. Interested specialists gather at conferences to deliberate the evidence. They form expert panels to flesh out the criteria for a given condition, to divide it into subtypes, to decide how best to test for and treat it.

Sometimes these diagnoses are listed, and so popularised, in diagnostic classification manuals (from the WHO or the American Psychiatric Association (APA), for example) and sanctioned by credible medical bodies such as the Royal College of Medicine or the US Centers for Disease Control and Prevention (CDC). These manuals may be used by researchers and medics around the world in training and diagnosing, and in developing treatments. There are caveats to this illusion of medical consensus, though: some diagnoses are contentious despite their appearance in international diagnostic manuals and mainstream academic journals. For example, the WHO recently classified gaming disorder as a condition of addictive behaviour, provoking significant criticism and consternation. More than two dozen international clinicians and researchers wrote an open letter stating that the disorder 'should be removed to avoid a waste of public health resources as well as to avoid causing harm to healthy video gamers around the world'.

The sociologist Annemarie Jutel has written that every diagnosis is a 'social creation'. 'That doesn't mean that the diseases it labels aren't "real", but it does mean that before a diagnosis can exist, it has to be visible, problematic, and perceived to be related to the field of medicine.'

Because diagnoses are, by definition, constructed, they are permeable to external influences. Diagnosis is supposed to offer us certainty: based in science, it should be free from sectarianism and uncomplicated by political or financial influence. Yet diagnostic labels are vulnerable to encircling biases and beliefs, despite the solid evidence base that seemingly cements their validity, despite the hard-won consensus that shapes their design. It befits us all to question who gets to publish their findings in mainstream journals, who takes part in international consensus meetings, who decides what goes into the diagnostic manuals and who controls the outcomes that flow from a diagnosis – and to note that what is often conspicuously absent is the voices of patients themselves. As an anonymous author once wrote, some people 'think they are thinking when they are merely rearranging their prejudices.'

We frequently, unconsciously, fall into the trap of seeing diagnosis as a universal appeal to truth. But in diagnosis there lies the danger of imagining, constructing, even fabricating a label to fit a narrative already written.

In this book we will meet the people who have incontrovertibly become patients through their medical diagnoses. But I'll interrogate whether this is a diagnostic delusion of sorts: when we lose our grip on the real purposes and applications of diagnosis, are we creating imaginary patients – people who should never be such, their agency diminished as a result of a diagnosis? Are we guilty of rupturing the patient's trust, of failing to listen and observe, of breaking the Hippocratic Oath, which rests on the tenet that one should 'do no harm'? Diagnosis is valuable and critical, and often delivered with good intentions; this book is therefore not an indictment of the medical establishment, although we will explore the delusions that have coloured its actions when they appear. Rather, it is frequently those outside the medical establishment who grievously leverage the power of diagnosis – the families of patients, the church, and the commercial companies that hover in the background.

Traditionally, we imagine that people are turned into

patients by the pharmaceutical industry, with its enthusiasm for offering potions and pills and remedies for everyday anxieties or imperceptibly receding hairlines. But what if there is something else going on at the heart of medicine? What if one of its most fundamental tools is implicated in the worst injustices of all?

In the stories that follow, we will hear from those who have borne diagnoses shaped by bias. Our imaginary patients are civil rights activists, gay men, asylum seekers, even babies not yet born. The prejudiced attitudes and actions they face are afforded a veneer of acceptability once a diagnosis is endorsed by the medical establishment. Perhaps the most perilous consequence is the egregious medical interventions to which the diagnosed have at times been subjected. Take one diagnosis made in the 1960s, in the former Soviet Union: political dissidents were imprisoned under the pretext that they were suffering from 'sluggish schizophrenia'. The characteristic signs of the condition included the expression of politically unacceptable views and 'reformist delusions'. Sluggish schizophrenia seemingly warranted the use of heavy-duty psychoactive drugs, imprisonment and solitary confinement.

Later, we will meet Jeremy, whose experience also exemplifies the way that diagnoses can sanction zealous medical intervention. He'll tell me about how the psychiatric diagnosis of homosexuality led to the electric shock aversion therapy treatment that he received in the 1970s and which almost brought him to the point of taking his own life.

The kind of partiality that can inform how diagnoses are made and the treatment that flows from them is a pressing concern of our time: children labelled with so-called behavioural disorders are being criminalised; teenagers diagnosed with putative brain disorders are being subjected to invasive and potentially lethal treatments; black men killed by law enforcement are being labelled with a condition that can serve to exonerate their murderers in the courts. All of these diagnoses have been backed recently by prominent and pre-eminent medical organisations.

But now is also an opportune time to intervene. You do not need to be a doctor; it may even be better if you are not. Medicine has been traditionally marked by paternalism, but now groups who have been too long under-represented are demanding change in all kinds of arenas. We all have an opportunity to speak out, to act, to protect. If we can comprehend the inherent flaws of diagnosis, we can begin that journey.

To understand how we got here, and to understand how we might shape the future, this book first examines the past. As I've mentioned, we tend to believe that diagnoses are fixed across time and space, but in fact diagnoses, even once formalised, do not inevitably endure. They are refined over time, often in line with new scientific discoveries, and sometimes disappear. We open with some transformative diagnoses of the nineteenth century, a period when the concept of diagnosis was rapidly evolving. Until then, illnesses had frequently been framed in descriptive terms, but over time a more formal listing of diseases developed, partly influenced by the demands of the new formalised system of death registration that began in the 1830s. The records of registered deaths soon included diagnoses more familiar to us today, including cholera, measles, epilepsy and diabetes. Many cases of what had been known as consumption (wasting) were relabelled as tuberculosis. Jail fever, found to be louse-borne, became typhus. An illness was deemed to be a disease, and a distinct diagnosis could then be delivered.

Even the diagnoses that in their day spawned thousands of scholarly papers, launched hundreds of medical conferences, made international headlines each week, or became the common currency of ward rounds in hospitals all over the world, could, as it turned out, be subject to revision.

Take 'devil's hair', also known as plica polonica. First described in the sixteenth century and later said to be endemic to Poland and Lithuania, it was characterised by an irreversibly matted mass of entangled hair. These plaits could 'reach the size of a large hat, or dangle from head to waist in one or several locks', becoming 'entangled as a hard stony mass resembling a bird's nest'. Some believed plica was the result of a witch's spell or a contagious supernatural occurrence. Regardless of its cause, plica polonica was said to provoke blindness, shrinkage of the arms and legs, convulsions, decay of the bones and paralysis. Treatment was complicated by the paradoxical belief of some people that a plait protected them from disease – they occasionally created one by drowning uncombed hair in wax, tar, resin and moss. There had been some nine hundred publications on plica polonica by the middle of the nineteenth century, and it inspired academic meetings across Europe solely devoted to that diagnosis.

Eventually, doctors realised it was a manifestation of seborrhoea – greasy, inflamed skin – of the same sort that contributes to dandruff. Late nineteenth-century medical literature categorically related the condition to a simple and rather unexciting neglect of one's hair.

Another disappeared diagnosis is chlorosis, which existed for some four hundred years. The Renaissance doctor who first described it in 1554 proposed a remedy: 'I instruct virgins afflicted with the disease that as soon as possible they live with men and copulate, if they conceive they recover.' The disease declared itself in young women with menstrual disturbances, melancholy, constipation, dizziness, lassitude, an appetite that could be 'capricious or depraved' and – as its name suggests – a green complexion to the skin. It was common, accounting for 6.1% of 3,001 attendances at Finsbury Dispensary, on the boundary of the City of London, by 1800. By 1900, the condition was beginning to fade a little, although there was mention of it in the medical literature for at least a couple of decades more. Its dissolution has been variably linked to improved nutrition, an increased understanding of female anatomy and the suffragette movement. Some women with these symptoms might in our time be diagnosed with an eating disorder or depression, which is not to say that these conditions are synonymous with chlorosis.

Both these conditions show how diagnostic labels represent a construction of sorts, influenced by the social and political environment in which they emerge. Plica polonica was imbued with prejudice and xenophobia, its descriptions often marked by references to interlopers and outsiders. Its cause was ascribed to 'the Mongol invasion' in medieval times, and later it was repeatedly described as a disease affecting only Jewish people – the *Juden-Zopff* (Jewish plait), some called it – that had made its way to London, 'brought over by the traders in false hair from Poland', and rendering 'its victim an object as hideous to behold as the lepers of the East'. Chlorosis was also shaped by cultural influences, steeped in and sculpted by a moral framework with patriarchal signatures. As late as 1916, a Valencian medical text advised: 'Sensationalist novels and unhealthy literature of all kinds should be absolutely prohibited. Girls should be spared intensive physical labour; they should be appropriately dressed, without the respiratory and circulatory obstructions imposed by modern corsets.'

Even if diagnoses remain, they are hardly stable, static or timeless. What was once borderline hypertension became, straightforwardly, hypertension when the threshold for a high blood pressure was lowered. The criteria for polycystic ovarian syndrome have likewise shifted over the last two decades, with some studies estimating a trebling or quadrupling of the number of diagnoses in women of reproductive age; and a new or mutated virus can bring a previously unknown pandemic to our shores with a corresponding diagnosis that declares itself in its millions.

Diagnoses old and new are not consistent geographically. Two patients may share similar clinical features and biological markers, but where they are can influence how these are labelled. Amnesia and dissociation (a disconnected feeling of not quite being located in your body and your surroundings) are interpreted as a spirit possession with healing properties by devotees of the Candomblé religion in north-eastern Brazil, while this sort of dissociation might be framed as 'multiple personality disorder' in North America or Europe. To acknowledge the profound complexities of characterising these diagnoses, their susceptibility to external influences and their worldwide variation is not to invalidate them or say they are 'made up'.

One fruitless question to ask of any diagnosis is whether it is 'real' or not. This question is predictably followed by a reductive and exhaustive search for a definitive physical marker or a typical biological signature. Finding either hallmark does not guarantee the existence of a diagnosis, nor does it always dismiss it. A diagnosis of chlorosis was once endorsed by its supporting clinical features ('perverted cravings for such things as coffee beans', ran one description). In the case of the so-called diagnosis of homosexuality, endless studies between the 1950s and 1990s declared that this 'psychiatric disorder' was associated with a definite level of this hormone or a distinct deficit of that one. Diagnoses can exist without definitive biological markers – in anxiety, there is no single brain region that is indisputably aberrant, no blood test irregularity that proves its presence. Neither of these truths invalidates the diagnosis or the suffering experienced by those with the condition. Equally, the mere unveiling of a biological signature does not make an entity pathological. If I unearth the neurobiological components of altruism or falling in love, that does not transform these things into diseases and then into diagnoses.

It is more useful to think about what these labels *do* to or for us. Whether they are helpful or harmful, whether they see us met with disbelief or acceptance, and how they shape the stories we tell – of ourselves and of others.

Let's return to Mrs Adebayo for a moment. Her diagnosis of Parkinson's meant that I was able to draw her symptoms together, explaining why she felt as she did. I could arrange a targeted test – a dedicated scan that searches for a deficit in dopamine. She and I could discuss treatment options – whether specialised physiotherapy for Parkinson's, or a medication that replenishes the depleted dopamine characteristic of the condition, or a targeted surgical treatment called deep brain stimulation, which sends electrical pulses to the brain regions that are disrupted in Parkinson's. We could discuss prognosis, because researchers have brought together people with the same diagnosis, observed their trajectory and published the findings. Mrs Adebayo could seek out support groups for those with the diagnosis and advocate for herself and others with it. It potentially legitimised and sanctioned her condition of being unwell – she could seek support or allowances at work, and she might qualify for disability benefits. A diagnosis imparted means a disease acknowledged. It is the cornerstone of trust between patient and doctor – you listened, you identified this condition, let us move forwards together from here.

But the absolute existence of Parkinson's as such seems unrelated to politics, religion, race, gender or sexuality. We might have yet to recognise its manifestations in their entirety. With time, research may split the condition into different subtypes. There is room to improve our treatments, and a pressing need to find a definitive cure. Nevertheless, its presence per se seems spared by the governing forces that inform some of the diagnoses I discuss in this book. Some of those are more obviously controversial and contested, marked by debate and dissent, yet others are perceived to be axiomatic and are roundly accepted; it takes some effort to peel back the layers of partiality, and to uncover, beneath, the experiences of those individuals living with these labels.

The consequences of applying a diagnostic label that is vulnerable to external biases are transformative, often in negative ways. Diagnoses can be used as instruments of social and political control; as value judgements; to legitimise ruthless or unsafe treatments; and to define a community, with lingering effects, as I'll learn when I visit the scene of the Handsworth riots of the 1980s. There, media reported on drug-addled delirious 'ganja junkies' with their 'Zulu-style war cries', and the press, police and medical establishment invoked the frequently imposed diagnosis of cannabis psychosis to characterise or condemn the actions of protestors.

In recent times a diagnosis predicament has emerged – a surge of diagnosis influencers with vested interests. The label of 'excited delirium' has been used to account for deaths under restraint, as the family of a Birmingham man who died at a police station will tell me. Through Mikey Powell's story, I'll explore how law enforcement, commercial enterprises and forensic medicine have nurtured and championed a diagnosis that critics say confuses and even conceals the true cause of death. In schools, a diagnosis called oppositional defiant disorder is being used to label children – primarily boys who are black – as hostile, enraged and defiant. What are the future ramifications of such a diagnosis for these children, and can we justify the diagnostic path we have taken? At a refugee camp on the Greek island of Lesbos, I'll meet a nine-year-old girl, Ayesha, from Afghanistan, who has been diagnosed with PTSD. It's an experience that will leave me questioning the essence of what diagnosis hopes to achieve. I'll also discover how commercial companies are mapping our genetic destinies, throwing us into a liminal space where we are not entirely well, but not unwell either.

And yet, if we reject contentious diagnostic labels wholesale, we risk undermining the struggle that some sufferers embark upon to receive a diagnosis. Some diagnosis influencers are patients themselves, and their families. I'll meet parents who are fighting for their child's controversial diagnostic label to be recognised, fighting for validation, authentication, research and the most effective treatment.

By exposing the often hidden networks that influence diagnosis, I believe we can address past injustices and prevent future ones. By challenging the prevailing orthodoxy around the infallibility of diagnosis, we can ultimately ensure that patients are met with the care and compassion they deserve.

At the heart of this account are the diagnosed – we'll encounter Jeremy, Sarah, Ayesha, Haseeb, Lucas, Finn and many others whose experiences, above all, inform what follows. I am grateful to them all for sharing their stories.

The Rise and Rise of Medicine

No topic more occupied the Victorian mind than Health [...]. In the name of Health, Victorians flocked to the seaside, tramped about in the Alps or Cotswolds, dieted, took pills, sweated themselves in Turkish baths, adopted this 'system' of medicine or that [...]. Victorians worshiped the goddess Hygeia, sought out her laws, and disciplined themselves to obey them.

The Healthy Body and Victorian Culture, Bruce Haley

The Victorians' obsession with the body extended to everything that could go awry with it. Their burgeoning enthusiasm for potions and pills, for care and cure, was welcomed by a medical establishment ready to decipher their ailments. Biting at the doctors' heels, though, were the quacks – allegedly contemptible, disreputable and medically unskilled peripatetic businessmen whose stock-in-trade was lurid advertisements and dishonest testimonials. These charlatans peddled elixirs and balsams that were at best redundant, and at worst deadly. In truth though, quacks, despite lacking a formal medical education, often offered similar syrups and even surgeries to those sold by orthodox medics, quoted the same legitimate scientific experts and listed themselves in the same medical directories (albeit under aliases or by stealing the names of dead doctors). In this unregulated system, the line between the two groups was indistinct, and accordingly there was much at stake: if trained doctors could secure the loyalty of seaside-flocking, Cotswolds-tramping, health-fixated Victorians, their standing would be elevated, and their scientific acumen asserted. There was money to be made too – this was not an aspiration limited to quacks.

At first glance, the medical establishment had little to recommend it over the nostrum vendors and potion pushers. At this time, the nation's health was bolstered more by improved social conditions – sanitation, housing and nutrition – than by groundbreaking cures. Tuberculosis still killed around one in five people in the early nineteenth century across Europe, and more people in Britain died from it between 1848 and 1872 than from any other disease. Cholera epidemics scarred the century, killing between 20,000 and 30,000 people across Britain in the 1831–2 outbreak alone. The public rioted against doctors accused of killing cholera patients to provide corpses to anatomists. It was not a baseless allegation; in 1828 in Edinburgh, William Burke and William Hare sold the bodies of their murder victims – numbering at least sixteen, perhaps many more – for medical dissection. Hare was let off after giving evidence against Burke at trial. Burke was executed for his crimes, and publicly dissected by an anatomist.

But the medical establishment had scientific progress on its side. Radical discoveries were being witnessed by a rapt public. Newfangled anaesthetics used by qualified medical practitioners, alongside Joseph Lister's pioneering antiseptic techniques, were revolutionising surgery. Queen Victoria received chloroform for the births of Prince Leopold in 1853 and Princess Beatrice in 1857 (the queen reported 'great relief from the vapour' and that it was 'delightful beyond measure'), a fact reported some years later in *The Times* under the headline 'Chloroform at the royal accouchement'.

Doctors were also developing an unprecedented understanding of infectious diseases like yellow fever, leprosy and cholera. In 1876, a specific bacterium (*Bacillus anthracis*) was, for the first time, shown by the German physician and microbiologist Robert Koch to cause a specific disease (anthrax). In 1885, a nine-year-old boy from Alsace who had been bitten by a rabid dog received a rabies vaccine from Louis Pasteur. The boy survived. Within five months, Pasteur wrote, patients were 'rushing here from England, Russia, Hungary, Italy and Germany. I would love to stop, but it is impossible'.* His successful anthrax inoculation experiments were relayed to London through daily dispatches from a *Times* reporter. By the end of the century, the bacterium responsible for bubonic plague had been discovered by the Pasteur-trained scientist Alexandre Yersin, and vaccination against smallpox had become standard practice.

The medical establishment was in the ascendency, and the diagnostic label was a potent tool in its assertion of supremacy. In the Age of Enlightenment, botanical classification systems for plants were enthusiastically expanded and repurposed for the organisation of diseases based on symptoms. In the nineteenth century, these systems were refined through anatomical, physio-logical and pathological discoveries. Cause seemingly could be linked to consequence – a revelatory lesion discovered on autopsy or a microorganism detected under a microscope could explain a patient's disease and direct scientists towards a cure.

Encircled by quacks as well as homeopaths, botanicals, wise

---

* Analysis of Pasteur's laboratory notebooks by the Princeton historian Gerald Geison suggests that the scientist used vaccines developed by collaborators but claimed these successes as his own. Pasteur also overstated the success of his previous experiments and reported that his vaccines had been thoroughly tested when they had not. See P. Allen, 'Pasteur's life and pioneering work', *Lancet*, 360/9326 (2002): 93.

women and druggists, the medical establishment championed three diagnoses in order to face down their detractors and cement its status: the first, spermatorrhea, distinguished medical professionals from quacks, or so the establishment claimed; the second, status lymphaticus, saw them attempt to explain a wave of sudden deaths in children; and the third, neurasthenia, did no less than encapsulate the modern post-industrial era. All three diagnoses have since disappeared in their original incarnations, which would have been almost unthinkable at the time, given the terror they evoked in their victims and the weight assigned to them by the establishment. Spermatorrhea was called one of 'the most dire, excruciating and deadly maladies to which the human frame is subject'. Status lymphaticus was labelled 'the most important problem in medicine'. Neurasthenia spread, plague-like, across the globe, threatening not only individuals but national identities too. Some historical diagnoses deserve to be consigned to the footnotes of medical texts, but not these ones. The medical establishment was shaped by them, for better or for worse. Their reverberations can still be felt today.

The diagnostic label of spermatorrhea – or excessive discharge of semen – owes its existence to Claude François Lallemand, Professor of Clinical Surgery at the University of Montpellier. Lallemand had identified the condition in one of his patients and was dismayed to find it remained resolutely refractory to his treatment of choice: the application of leeches to the man's anus. Much later, when he performed an autopsy of the same patient, who had seemingly died from his seminal incontinence, he noticed that one of the man's testicles was larger than the other. This, Lallemand decided, was a crucial hallmark of spermatorrhea. It was a disease, Lallemand wrote, 'that degrades man, poisons the happiness of his best days, and ravages society'.

Masturbation was inevitably blamed – although any illicit or excessive sexual activity would do. There was a litany of precipitating factors: soft beds, flannel trousers, sleeping on one's back and thunderstorms. 'One unfortunate soul ejaculated twice on the Brighton–London train because he sat instead of standing.' The affliction formally became a medical concern, and a diagnosis, through Lallemand's writings; his three-volume *Des Pertes Séminales Involontaires* ('On involuntary seminal loss') was published between 1836 and 1842.

But excessive ejaculation was not a novel concern, even if spermatorrhea became a particular preoccupation of the Victorian era. Anxiety around semen loss was explored in Ayurvedic texts between the fifth millennium BC and the seventh century AD, and the potentially alarming consequences of masturbation were summarised by the Greek physician and philosopher Galen (129–c. 216): 'No normal man might actually become a woman, but each man trembled forever on the brink of becoming "womanish".'

Lallemand's work, even if its concepts were of its time, spoke to a receptive public in an era in which masturbation was a particular moral and social concern. Sexual deviations, once linked to religious invocations of wickedness and demonic possession, had been reframed in the eighteenth century as threats to health. In the bestselling book *Onania*, published around 1710, an anonymous author wrote of the physical consequences of masturbation: 'Men, who were strong and lusty before they gave themselves over to this vice, have been wore out by it, and by its robbing the body of its balmy and vital moisture, without cough or spitting, dry and emaciated, sent to their Graves'.

The message of *Onania* was amplified by the celebrated Swiss physician and devout Calvinist Samuel Tissot, in another bestselling and highly influential book published in 1758 (the first English translation appeared in 1766). In *L'Onanisme* (*Onanism*),

Tissot brought a scientific narrative to bear alongside a moral one: masturbation increased blood flow, which weakened the nerves, leaving them 'enfeebled'. These fears around the putative consequences for health chimed with wider Enlightenment and Protestant ideas about policing and controlling the mind and imagination, and with changing perceptions of the body and masculine selfhood in the eighteenth century. There were plenty of vested commercial interests willing to capitalise on these concerns.

Spermatorrhea, as described by Lallemand, made its way into popular pamphlets and medical textbooks alike. Nocturnal and diurnal emissions, premature ejaculation and impotence were characteristic. Disturbing and disfiguring effects became well known. Misfortunate sufferers were abruptly struck by a bloated and blotchy face with dark circles under the eyes, baldness and 'whiskers and beard stunted in growth'. The British physician and clergyman's son Dr William Acton described the permanent effects of spermatorrhea on the 'timbre of the voice', as well as a debilitating hoarseness and dryness of the throat. Acton's recommended cure? Victims should desist from 'titillation and friction of the virile member with the hand'. This was a condition of the mind too: patients were enveloped by melancholy, tearfulness, loss of confidence and profound amnesia.

The emergence of the diagnosis was equally convenient for the medical establishment. Here were patients plagued with deep-rooted concerns about their masculinity, their minds and their morals. They needed help, they sought help, and if the medical establishment didn't intervene, the charlatans already circling them surely would. Medicine's scathing view of these quacks was encapsulated in a *Lancet* editorial in the 1850s, which denounced them as 'men who have sacrificed science and debased morality, embracing falsehood and practising deception'. Quackery was, the editorial continued, 'the curse of the age [...] the growing vice of modern society, the canker in the bud of our progress'. No doubt there were many well-meaning and skilled medics who wished to help and heal their patients. It's unlikely, however, that the chance of professional advancement went unnoticed, nor did the calibre of clientele – the condition was considered one of middle-class men,* and so could command lucrative income.

Could the medical establishment step in instead of the quacks, see off these pretenders and emerge as the righteous victor? In laying claim to the diagnosis of spermatorrhea much was at stake, and both sides were ready for a fight. The battleground: a museum in central London owned by a purported quack, filled with waxworks of body organs and monstrosities in jars.

Dr Joseph Kahn's Anatomical and Pathological Museum was located first at 315 Oxford Street, then the Salle Robin at 232 Piccadilly. Early medical opinions of the museum were glowing. Writing in the *Lancet*, doctors in the early 1850s marvelled at the 'microscopical figures' that showed 'the progress of the ovum in the uterus from the time impregnation takes place to birth', and the life-sized Anatomical Venus 'which takes [*sic*] to pieces for the purpose of exposing the general anatomy and the relations of the various viscera [...]. Altogether it is a splendid scientific collection, and a great deal of general information is to be obtained by a visit'.

However, there is no concrete evidence that Kahn held authentic medical credentials, even though he described himself as a 'medical doctor' in the census. The museum was highly profitable, as was the venereal disease clinic he ran alongside it: 'He rented a large

---

* Ellen Rosenman, Emeritus Professor of English at the University of Kentucky, believes this was because these were men who 'tended to postpone the legitimate sexual outlet of marriage until they were financially secure, they were prey to sexual panic because of class-specific constraints on erotic pleasure, and they could afford medical care' (*Unauthorized Pleasures*, 2018).

house in Harley Street,' writes pathologist Alan William Bates, and 'furnished it lavishly, kept a carriage and pair, and rode in the park.'

The *Handbook of Dr. Kahn's Museum*, provided free to visitors, listed a dizzying array of spermatorrhea symptoms: 'erections and emissions upon slightest excitement', 'cadaverous appearance of skin', 'pimples on shoulders and forehead', 'hollow or sunken eyes', and 'strange or lascivious dreams'. Here are the descriptions of some of the nine anatomical models detailing the condition in the handbook:

> 1175: Atrophy, or diminution of the prostrate and penis, caused by indulgence in the odious vice of Onanism.
> 1178: Spermatorrhea caused by the irritation produced by ascarides (worms) in the anus.
> 1180: Spermatorrhea – a few drops of seminal fluid passing from the urethra after the expulsion of the urine.
> 1183: Spermatorrhea – efflux of blood following expulsion of urine in a case where Onanism had been practised to a very great extent.

There was even a section called 'Self-Diagnosis' – a doctor was barely needed at all.

Anatomical museums in Victorian times provided education, sometimes of the moral sort, and entertainment for the public, and Kahn's, complete with its calamitous warnings around masturbation and spermatorrhea, welcomed thousands of visitors each month. In 1853, the *Lancet* recorded that the museum had received 'golden opinions from all sorts of people', including 'the leading medical men of Scotland and Ireland'. And yet, in contrast, a letter published in the same journal just a few years later read: 'So disgusting and immoral, so determinedly arranged for the purposes of depraving the minds of the ignorant and unwary, are the contents of this place, that their public exhibition should be suppressed by those who pretend to guard public morals and to respect public decency.'

Why such a remarkable volte-face? It was a matter of reputation. By 1857, legislation was emerging that sought to distinguish qualified from unqualified practitioners. A succession of writers to the *Lancet* that year called for action against 'imposters, rogues, charlatans and quacks' and their 'explicit' and 'revolting' pamphlets and displays. Commercial museums were fast becoming the subject of disdain among medics who realised they needed to be viewed as clinicians of repute rather than curators of obscenity. Kahn had, they claimed, privileged earnings over education and monstrosities over medicine. He and his contemporaries were charged with preying 'with a relentless and vulture-like rapacity' upon their victims through 'pseudo-scientific lectures', 'specious advertisements' and 'dirty and filthy handbills'.

In truth, writes the historian Elizabeth Stephens, there was sometimes little to distinguish museums like Kahn's from 'respectable' medical museums. The Hunterian Museum, Stephens writes, 'contained exhibits such as a comparative display of the skeletons of the "Irish Giant," Charles Byrne, and the "Sicilian Fairy," Caroline Crachami, that would not be out of place in a commercial venue such as Kahn's.' Yet the Hunterian was originally the private collection of the British surgeon and anatomist John Hunter, later purchased by the government for £15,000 and presented to the Company (later Royal College) of Surgeons in London in 1799. It was open to medical men and scientists, as well as select elites: peers, 'great officers of state', church dignitaries and flag officers.

The reality behind the resistance of some physicians and surgeons, or at least the depth of their resistance, might instead have lain in the threat that these public museums, with their accompanying clinics and quack remedies, posed to the establishment. Those outraged letters to the *Lancet* were penned just months after the formation of the British Medical Association (BMA) – previously the Provincial Medical and Surgical Association – with its keen ambition for medical reform. As those letters made their way into print, transformative medical legislation was also being introduced, cemented by the Medical Act 1858, which finally provided qualified practitioners with statutory recognition. The General Medical Council (GMC) was established to register qualified practitioners, monitor standards of professional training and deregister practitioners guilty of criminal acts or 'infamous conduct in any professional respect'. A victory against Kahn and his contemporaries might now also restore the reputation of medical men, who were often characterised at the time, as the historian Terry Parssinen writes, as 'a profession filled with marginal men: drunken, randy medical students; 'half-caste' army and navy surgeons; impecunious Scots with dubious medical degrees in their kits; and irreligious professors of anatomy who furtively purchased exhumed corpses from graverobbers.' The deep opposition to the Kahn museum, then, was steeped in the ambitions and aspirations of the medical profession. Anatomical exhibits should be their territory. So too should the diagnosis of spermatorrhea.

It was in the condition's treatment that surgeons, even more so than physicians, could differentiate themselves from swindlers and medical impostors – a rebranding of sorts, even if it may not have been a conscious pursuit of professionalisation. Until now, surgeons had occupied the middle tier between the more prestigious physicians and the lower-ranked apothecaries (who made and dispensed medications). Physicians were educated at elite universities in the classics rather than exposed to cadavers. Surgeons underwent technical apprenticeships instead. While physicians received honoraria, surgeons could set their fees, which aligned them with tradesmen.

By 'owning' spermatorrhea, surgeons could attempt to cast off their reputation as barbers and manual labourers and, in the words of Professor Ellen Rosenman, 'enrich their cultural capital'. As the doors of the supposedly obscene museums closed, patients diagnosed with spermatorrhea could instead be wheeled through the open doors of an operating theatre where a qualified surgeon was waiting, ready to intercede.

But the Medical Act had not succeeded in outlawing quacks, since it only regulated qualified practitioners; quacks could simply continue unregistered. The medical establishment had another tactic to counter this. Several anatomy museums were prosecuted under the Obscene Publications Act 1857, vigorously endorsed by the evangelical Society for the Suppression of Vice, and financed by none other than the Quack Prosecution Fund, a group of medical practitioners.

The polemics against Kahn's work succeeded – first the museum temporarily shut its doors in 1858, then he faced prosecution for unlicensed practice (but left the country before the case came to pass). Proceedings against the museum rumbled on, and in 1873 its then owners pleaded guilty to offences under the Obscene Publications Act and a magistrate ordered that the stock be destroyed. Mr Collette, prosecuting solicitor for the Society for the Suppression of Vice, was granted permission to strike the first blow: 'Accompanied by Police Inspector Harnett and Sergeant Butcher, he proceeded to smash with a hammer the first of the anatomical waxes, the fragments of which were then handed back to the defendants.'

Other public anatomy museums also faced opprobrium and were prosecuted under the Obscene Publications Act, including, in 1860, Louis Lloyd's anatomical museum in Leeds, and Joseph

Woodhead's anatomical museum in Manchester, which was closed
by the police in 1874.

Spermatorrhea was energetically leveraged as a diagnosis that
allowed valiant doctors to save patients from unscrupulous and
unlicensed swindlers. But the medical establishment now needed
to appropriate the diagnosis whose treatment it coveted.

The first step in any diagnostic landgrab is to medicalise
it – in other words, to use a medical framework to understand
and treat a problem. So doctors duly set to publishing autopsy
results on spermatorrhea sufferers and used microscopy to detect
spermatozoa in the urine – a process technically possible since
the seventeenth century, but increasingly used from the 1850s
onwards.

After investigation, there was treatment. Willing, or perhaps
frantic, patients lined up. Dr Kahn frequently published letters
from self-declared spermatorrhea sufferers:

> I am twenty-seven years of age, of a delicate, nervous
> temperament; I am single, and likely to remain so, unless
> you can assist me; for there is no disguising the fact, I am
> impotent through the effects of self-pollution.

And another, who admitted practising 'the degrading vice of
self-abuse':

> The fact of being engaged to an amiable and
> accomplished young lady whom I had [sic] known
> several years, coupled with the terrible, fearful thoughts
> of impotency, drives me almost wild. As a Christian, and
> one who I believe has the welfare of his fellow men at
> heart, I beseech you to do what you can to restore some
> of my former vigour […] I have given up, and for ever,

the vile practice that has been draining away my life's
blood. God grant it may (through your help) not be
too late.

First-line treatments were relatively benign: gymnastics, a brisk
walk, banishing impure thoughts, sponging with cold salt water,
perhaps a suppository or two. But if these failed, eye-watering
techniques awaited, which surgeons asserted they were singularly
qualified to conduct. Most surgeons who treated spermatorrhea
advocated chemical irritants, including the British surgeon John
Laws Milton, who used the technique of cauterisation – a metal
instrument inserted through the urethra, coated with a caustic
agent such as silver nitrate or mercury to deaden the nerves: '[C]
auterisation has rarely failed to give more or less relief [...]. Of its
safety there can be no doubt' (despite violent spasms in patients
and reportedly even deaths). He also recommended that patients
wear a spiked metal 'urethral ring' and an electric alarm that would
sound at the first sign of a nocturnal erection, inducing blisters
to the penis. The US surgeon Robert Bartholow encouraged
injections of cold water into the rectum in addition to 'nitrate
of silver, sulphate of copper, acetate of lead', but also praised the
success of anal dilation:

> I have had excellent results from stretching the sphincter
> ani. The method as pursued by me consists in the
> introduction of a bi-valve rectal speculum, and then
> working the screw until the blades are sufficiently
> separated. The operation causes considerable pain, and
> may rupture the sphincter if incautiously carried too far.

Some dissenters did emerge. In 1871, the surgeon George G.
Gascoyen told the medical Harveian Society of London that

Lallemand's book was 'a striking example of how an able man can mislead himself when he has a theory to prove'. Sir James Paget thought spermatorrhea might have been a Frenchman's sickness but was surely 'unknown among Englishmen'. Despite concerns expressed by these sceptics, it was taken seriously by the mainstream medical profession for several decades.

Later in the nineteenth century, surgical interest in the condition of spermatorrhea began to wane. Reconstructed as a disease of the mind, 'over-sensitive nervous systems' and 'defects of will' were now implicated. Catheterisation and cold enemas were nevertheless still frequently recommended. The condition disappeared from the *Nomenclature of Diseases* by the 1920s, but public fear regarding the effects of spermatorrhea persisted, and it continued to feature in popular books such as *Harmsworth's Home Doctor & Encyclopaedia of Good Health*.*

Despite the retreat of spermatorrhea, many in the nineteenth-century medical establishment, surgeons in particular, were much indebted to, of all things, a condition of seminal incontinence. By successfully staking claim to the diagnosis, they had cemented their status, disparaging quacks and public anatomy museums along the way.

Their ultimate ownership of the diagnosis reflected a broader cultural change that had seen their prominence and reputation grow – an increasing understanding of how diseases unfurl, the emergence of transformative vaccines and the evolution of medical treatments and surgical techniques. Even then, a single diagnosis such as spermatorrhea could not grant medics absolute

---

* Just because the diagnosis faded, it doesn't mean that concerns about seemingly excessive ejaculation have too. In the Indian subcontinent, for instance, anxiety around semen loss, termed 'dhat' from the Sanskrit (dhatu = metal, elixir) remains prevalent.

authority or exonerate them from criticism (in May 1894, for instance, the *Daily Chronicle* labelled their practices a form of 'human vivisection'); but when combined with the considerable medical advances of the age, the profession unquestionably achieved a more elevated status. What was more, in the nineteenth century, doctors for the first time went beyond their original mandate of diagnosing ailments among the living. From the mid-1830s, they were called upon to explain their demise too, in the form of a death certificate. A small piece of paper, perhaps, but a monumental step towards authority and agency. And yet, one of those explanations of death threatened the living. It would take decades for doctors to realise their mistake. Before they did so, an untold number of children would pay the price.

Understanding diseases of the living is prefigured by disentangling the mysteries of death. Autopsies shed light on the metastatic spread of a cancer, the trajectory of a stroke, the predilection of an infection for this organ or that. Death certificates act as a historical record of how we have come to define and diagnose disease.

In Europe from late medieval times right up to the beginning of the nineteenth century, recording cause of death served primarily religious and bureaucratic needs: to document basic sacramental requirements of Christian faith – baptism, marriage and burial – and for probating wills and testaments. It was the onslaught of bubonic plague that prompted systematic population-wide reporting of deaths for the first time. Civil death registers from Milan (the *Necrologi*) began in the fifteenth century and soon shaped how plague deaths were recorded in London.

Beginning from the 1592 plague, when they were issued sporadically, the London *Bills of Mortality* were published regularly from the early 1600s onwards – every Thursday, with a general overview of the year on the Thursday before Christmas Day.

They carried death figures from Anglican burials across the city's parishes on a single sheet of paper. Some of the 'diseases and casualties' listed seem prosaic ('cough', 'winde'); others are more unfamiliar to us today. 'King's evil' is believed to have represented scrofula, or a tubercular infection of the lymph glands in the neck, named for the belief that a touch from a monarch could cure it. In March 1684, six or seven people were 'prest and trod to death' at St Martin-in-the-Fields in a stampede to be touched for the condition. 'Rising of the lights' is thought have to have been a respiratory condition, possibly croup.

Occasionally, the descriptions were more dramatic, almost poetic: 'drowned at S[t] Kathar[ine's] Tower', 'griping in the Guts', 'found dead in the Street at Stepney', 'kil[le]d accidentally with a Carbine, at St Michael Woodstreet', 'scalded in a Brewers Mash at St Giles Cripplegate'.

These were gathered not by medical men, but by 'searchers', alerted to deaths in their own parishes. Searchers were older women, often widows, sometimes illiterate. They inspected the corpses of the dead and made a judgement on the final illness, reporting their findings to the parish clerk. Despite the absence of medical terminology, at least as we know it now, statisticians could track the spread of plague as well as determine the growth of the city, and collate the cost of its diseases. On a more practical basis, they informed daily life – playhouses could reopen, for instance, when plague deaths numbered fewer than 30 per week.

In contrast to the searchers, most medical men then in day-to-day practice were not employed to name specific diseases. Instead, they explained the *processes* underlying them – descriptive accounts of, for example, ulcerated lesions, hyperactive nerves and sexual excesses. Fluid gathered, blood congealed, passions mounted – a patient needed to be purged or bled or rested.

The Registration Act 1836 transformed this approach by making the state registration of births, marriages and deaths compulsory. It remained a bureaucratic and statistical endeavour rather than a medical one, established to accurately record lines of descent and establish property rights (the existing piecemeal system fell short of the task and was facing growing criticism as a result). There was a public health impetus too: statisticians and sanitarians believed the data could reveal which factors determined good, or poor, health.

The local registrar had to be notified of each death, with doctors providing a written statement explaining its cause. In 1845, the accuracy of the process was dialled up – the Registrar General provided specific forms for medical practitioners to fill out. A Royal College of Physicians (RCP) committee got on board, drawing up a classification of disease to aid this process. In 1874, the Births and Deaths Registration Act set out formal procedures for certification, with a penalty (40 shillings) for failure to deliver a medical certificate. Certification from a doctor was now needed before burial or cremation, and their expertise was also required to explain suspicious deaths. There was a slap on the wrist for sloppiness too – the Registrar General contacted practitioners when the wording on certificates was ambiguous. In 1860, 80% of registered deaths were certified by medical practitioners, rising to 97.7% by the end of the century.*

---

* To investigate 'sudden or unnatural' deaths, coroners did not have to be medical men – in the nineteenth century, most were solicitors and only 14% were medically qualified. However, the 1836 Medical Witness Act encouraged medical participation by providing payment for post-mortems and for giving evidence at inquests. The 1836 Registration Act required that inquests provide 'medically credible verdicts', thus elevating the importance of medical opinion. See G. H. H. Glasgow, 'The campaign for medical coroners in nineteenth-century England and its aftermath', *Mortality*, 9/2 (2004).

In 1875, William Farr, the first statistician at the General Register Office, wrote that 'the returns of the causes of death show that diagnosis, though still imperfect, has within 35 years made remarkable progress not only among the foremost physicians and surgeons of the day, but among the body of medical practitioners all over the kingdom who give certificates'. Farr was invited to draw up a classification system at the 1864 International Statistical Congress, which influenced systems of death registration worldwide.

There were still shortcomings, of course. Doctors occasionally avoided mention of 'socially sensitive' diseases such as syphilis, for the sake of grieving families. For women, a history of recent childbirth was sometimes omitted, which might have been a tactic by medical men to evade charges of incompetence or worse. But the authority of doctors had been firmly established, because now they were not only needed in life, but also in death.

Even if evolving registration requirements hadn't propelled doctors to explain deaths in the nineteenth century, another force soon would have. Increasingly, in the latter part of the century, children seemed to be dying suddenly – ominously – while in the hands of their doctors. Children undergoing even minor operations were losing their lives, and in mounting numbers. A new explanation for these terrible fatalities was needed, in Britain and further afield. The diagnosis that doctors landed upon – status lymphaticus – says much about how the medical establishment used diagnosis not only to explain death, but also to exonerate itself from accusations of manslaughter.

In Victorian Britain, children were vulnerable, and infants especially so. Around the middle of the century, a third of children under the age of five died, often succumbing to measles, whooping cough, scarlet fever, smallpox and diphtheria – compounded by malnourishment and poor sanitation.

Sudden deaths were more difficult to explain and yet an

explanation was crucial – not only for bereaved families but, in this new era of death registration, for practical reasons. In the seventeenth and eighteenth centuries, 'visitation of God' had frequently been cited by coroners, but in an era of secularisation and medicalisation this terminology would not do. In a parliamentary discussion of the Coroner's Bill, Lord Harry Vane observed that magistrates in Devon had decided that 'whenever the verdict of the coroner's jury in that county was "Died by the visitation of God", they should disallow the fees of the coroner'. Infant mortality rates were included in the Registrar General's annual report for the first time ever in 1877, reflecting the emergence of a social awareness of these deaths and, says sociologist David Armstrong, 'the social recognition of the infant as a discrete entity'. 'Visitation of God' failed as an explanation, especially so when a new condition seemed to be killing off children who had been taken to doctors to be helped, not harmed.

With hindsight, the cause seems simple. Decades beforehand, concerns had emerged about the growing use of chloroform for anaesthesia, especially in the hands of unskilled practitioners. In 1853 (the same year that Queen Victoria gave birth to a son with its aid), the *Lancet* reported on chloroform-related deaths: 'It is for ourselves a melancholy duty to record these unfortunate instances [...] chloroform takes away pain but it also takes away life.' In 1869, the *British Medical Journal* (*BMJ*) cautioned that chloroform was 'hardly to be recommended for general use'. Chloroform was not, however, widely implicated by doctors in the deaths of these children who had been operated on. Instead, some prominent figures in the medical establishment began to speculate that 'constitutional weakness' was to blame. The findings of a pathologist in Vienna named Arnold Paltauf conveniently appeared to support such a theory.

In 1889, Paltauf published the results of autopsies on five

of his patients – infants who had died suddenly in unknown circumstances, and young adults who had died suddenly while swimming. They shared signatures of constitutional weakness, he argued: an enlarged thymus (even though there were no standards for 'normal' thymus size at the time) and/or hyperplasia (a proliferation of cells) of all lymphoid tissues. This new diagnosis was labelled 'status lymphaticus'. The label was co-opted by those who sought to explain, perhaps justify, sudden deaths under chloroform. Cause (hyperplasia of the lymphoid tissues) and consequence (sudden death) were inextricably linked. Status lymphaticus was cited as causing hundreds of deaths in Britain each year. Across Europe and North America, the diagnosis was extended to explain the unexpected deaths of children after trivial stress or a sudden shock. The literature around status lymphaticus flourished – at least 820 academic papers were published in the three decades after it was first described – and it was researched by some of the most influential doctors of the time. With the advent of this new diagnosis, the potential dangers of chloroform were easily dismissed. In 1910, the BMA issued the *Final Report Of [the] Special Chloroform Committee*, stating that 'dangers arising from the status lymphaticus [...] are incidental to anaesthesia, and fall outside the range of the present report'.

As Ann Dally discovered in her extensive historical review of the condition, it became a matter of urgency to diagnose children in life, whether they were going for any sort of operation or not. Firstly, so that they could be treated before status lymphaticus killed them. And secondly and paradoxically, so that doctors could avoid manslaughter charges, as the *Lancet* warned, due to overdosing or the toxicity of anaesthetics in cases where status lymphaticus was thought to be present. The expertise of the medical establishment was vital to saving these children; its authority was sought and valued.

Children were diagnosed through X-rays (to assess the size of the thymus – a technique later shown to be grossly inaccurate) and physical examination. Doctors were taught to identify the typical features of a child with status lymphaticus: 'pale and pasty', 'flabby', and 'short-necked'. Douglas Symmers, a pathologist at Bellevue Hospital in New York, identified the condition in 6.2% of his autopsies, publishing his results in *The American Journal of Diseases of Children*: 'The face is beardless, or nearly so, and the axillary [armpit] and other hairs are scanty, the skin is smooth and unusually delicate, the pubic hairs are sharply defined in a transverse direction.' Status lymphaticus was more difficult to identify in females, wrote Symmers, but 'delicate skin, [a] narrow waist, and arched thighs' were supportive.

Children diagnosed with the condition had their thymus removed surgically – often under chloroform. A third of these children died.

At the beginning of the twentieth century, as status lymphaticus purportedly reached epidemic proportions, children diagnosed with the condition had radiation therapy to shrink the thymus instead of surgery to remove it, a procedure first carried out on an infant in the US, by Dr William H. Crane of Cincinnati in 1905. Crane and his colleague, Dr Friedlander, set up an X-ray machine in the child's home. They created a field for the radiation treatment by cutting a hole in tinfoil ('to the size of a silver dollar that the infant's father provided'). They deemed the treatment, delivered over several weeks, an unmitigated success, paving the way for others. Many more holes would be cut in sheets of tinfoil, and many more children would be irradiated.

The price paid by countless children would only become known later. In 1950 in New York, researchers discovered an irrefutable link between radiation treatment and cancer – thyroid cancer in children was 100 times more common in those who had received radiation treatment in early life. Yet radiation treatment for status lymphaticus was still championed years after that widely published New York study.

It was not only this cancer risk that was neglected in the excitement around a novel diagnosis, but also the simple explanation that chloroform was potentially fatal in the first place. In 1911, there were 276 deaths in England and Wales where anaesthesia was mentioned (in children and adults), and yet the Registrar General's report that year stated that '[I]t seems illogical to class deaths primarily to anaesthetics, since the primary cause must always be some condition which has occasioned the administration of an anaesthetic'. This was almost 60 years after the *Lancet* had recorded 'chloroform takes away pain but it also takes away life'. Of those 276 deaths, status lymphaticus was cited for 31. These conclusions continued to be drawn over the next decade. In England and Wales between 1911 and 1924, status lymphaticus was cited as cause of death under anaesthesia in up to around 300 children under the age of fifteen. The condition was listed as cause of death in about 200 patients each year who had not received anaesthetic.

So why was this obvious potential cause of children's deaths ignored? An unsettling motive might be this: general anaesthetics had transformed medicine and elevated the status of those who administered them. Chloroform was convenient — it was easy to administer, only required a small dose, and took effect rapidly. More ominously, only a small proportion of deaths under anaesthesia in private practice ever came to the attention of registrars or coroners. When deaths were reported, anaesthetists could strike back with a diagnosis that exonerated themselves. The dead had been constitutionally weak in life, they implied. The dead had no right of reply.

With time, the diagnosis of status lymphaticus came under sustained fire. A 1923 report from the Medical Research Council and the Pathological Society of Great Britain and Ireland rejected a link between an enlarged thymus and sudden death. X-rays could not reliably assess thymus size in children, and there were no standards for what the 'normal' thymus weighed, they concluded. The British researchers Major Greenwood and Hilda Woods characterised status lymphaticus as a 'heap of rubbish [...] treated as an orthodox shrine' and an example of 'medical mythology'. In 1931, the *Lancet* published an editorial called 'The end of status lymphaticus':

> It is simple humanity to search for some explanation
> which will satisfy the modem mind where the 'visitation
> of God' would once have been enough. Hence the
> doctrine of 'status lymphaticus' which, owing to our
> ignorance of the anatomy of the normal healthy human
> body, has survived longer than it should.

At first, not everyone was convinced. Preoperative radiotherapy was routinely administered to every child with a supposedly enlarged thymus who attended the Massachusetts Eye and Ear Hospital until 1940. In England, Alan Moncrieff, Professor of Child Health at the Hospital for Sick Children in Great Ormond Street (and medical correspondent for *The Times*), remained a proponent of both the diagnosis and the irradiation of the thymus gland, a treatment he continued to offer in the 1930s and beyond. The royal paediatrician Sir Wilfrid Sheldon included status lymphaticus in his 1943 textbook *Diseases of Infancy and Childhood*, which supported the use of radiation treatment until its eighth edition in 1962, over a decade after researchers confirmed an inextricable link between radiation treatment in childhood and thyroid cancer.

Few diagnoses die on scientific evidence alone, just as few diagnoses are shaped free of societal, cultural and political influences. Status lymphaticus arose in a perfect storm of increasing medicolegal concern, heightened anxiety about child health and scientific advances in radiology and anaesthetics. The diagnosis had faded by the 1970s, its own death hastened by restrictions around chloroform use, associations made between chloroform and heart failure, its replacement by other safer anaesthetics, and emergent explanations and descriptions for sudden deaths in children (unrelated to anaesthetic), such as anaphylaxis, sepsis and 'cot death' – later termed sudden infant death syndrome.

In its lifetime, status lymphaticus was symbolic of the almost unchallenged power and privilege that the medical establishment had carved out for itself. Through a novel diagnosis, in seemingly trying to save infants and children, some in the medical establishment had managed, above all, to save themselves.

Medicine, in its most potent form, crystallises not just how we are feeling but who we have become. Occasionally, a new diagnosis is emblematic of an era. Through the nineteenth century ailment of neurasthenia, medicine provided a means for people to make sense of their changing world. But neurasthenia carries a sinister history, one embroiled in colonial exceptionalism and eugenics. It was a condition that was considered highly desirable, until it became anything but.

Neurasthenia – a state of nervous exhaustion – was described in 1869 by the New York physician George Miller Beard as the plague of the modern age:* 'The chief and primary cause of this development and very rapid increase of nervousness is modern civilization, which is distinguished from the ancient by these five characteristics: steampower, the periodical press, the telegraph,

---

* Beard wasn't the first to use the term, but he was the first to define it in such detail, and popularised its use.

the sciences, and the mental activity of women.' This crushing 'want of strength in the nerve' saw sufferers overwhelmed by symptoms that emerged acutely or insidiously, and often lingered: incapacitating fatigue, headaches, palpitations, anxiety, downcast mood, indigestion, insomnia, widespread aches and pains, and sexual impotence.

Neurasthenia was a response to the stresses and strains of modern society, Beard explained – he had fallen victim to the condition himself. One's finite source of nervous energy was drained by the relentless pace of life, one's psyche assaulted by the onslaught of inventions and discoveries. These contemporary pressures permeated the atmosphere of modern civilisation like bacteria saturating the air, wrote one of Beard's contemporaries, inhaled by its unsuspecting citizens: 'Like the living microscopic germs, they make their easiest victims of those whose powers of resistance are weakest'. There was occasional moral fragility too – the profligate wastage of nerve force on promiscuity and gambling. On Sunday 28 December 1902, the neurasthenic novelist Theodore Dreiser wrote in his diary: 'Nervous condition rather worse this morning owing to a foolish hour of trifling with Mrs. D.'

Its casualties were many. The German sociologist Max Weber was afflicted, as were the philosopher and psychologist William James, the social reformer and writer Charlotte Perkins Gilman and the novelist Marcel Proust, even, in his youth, the US president Theodore Roosevelt. Neurasthenia entered the writings of Henry James, Jack London, Kate Chopin and Thomas Mann – as well as Edith Wharton, who wrote of how her husband's 'sweetness of temper and boyish enjoyment of life struggled long against the creeping darkness of neurasthenia'.

In truth, a novel disease had not arisen because of a changing world – but a novel diagnosis *did* help to decipher a time of tremendous social and cultural change. The condition emerged in the decades after the American Civil War, as migration from rural communities to urban ones gathered force – eleven million people in all between 1870 and 1920, joined in the cities by most of the twenty-five million immigrants arriving in the US. The country was transformed from a predominately rural agrarian society to an industrial economy centred in metropolitan cities. Farmers and tradesmen became businessmen and office workers. Women increasingly studied and worked outside the home. Some innovations emerged within the country, others were imported into it – all changed the face of a nation: assembly-line production and electrification, steam engines and skyscrapers, calculators and typewriters, telephones and telegraphs, escalators and rollercoasters.

Neurasthenia could assimilate cultural anxieties around these changing times into the health concerns of its sufferers – a businessman's new headaches as he strove for affluence, a woman's palpitations as she pursued academic excellence. It was a captivating and plausible diagnosis which allowed people to explain the world around them, and to explain themselves too, without wholly implicating or indicting their own inadequacies.

Many of those cultural anxieties resonate strongly today. Dr E. H. Van Deusen, in 1869, mourned 'the hot-house educational system of the present day', and a concerned physician, Dr Frederick MacCabe, wrote in 1875 that 'telegrams arriving at all hours with fluctuating quotations, and producing rapid alternations of hope and fear, must preclude all possibility of mental repose'. In 1881, George Beard noted that new appliances and technologies were 'the causes of noises that are unrhythmical, unmelodious and therefore annoying, if not injurious.'

Neurasthenia embedded itself within the medical community, its details filling hundreds of journal articles and textbooks in the late nineteenth century – one case series alone, published in 1899, listed 330 patients. Subtypes were identified (cerebral, gastric or genital). Instruments were manufactured to measure it. Specialist doctors emerged to treat it. Although neurasthenia traversed the social divide, Beard characterised it as a 'distinguished malady'; some doctors, as compassionate as they might have been, must have appreciated that many of their patients would be wealthy enough to afford repeated expensive consultations and treatments.

For some patients, complete physical and mental rest for up to three months was recommended, to restore energy through increasing the body's fat and blood, or so the theory went. This rest treatment was especially directed towards women, a not-so-subtle command to shuffle back to a state of passivity. Gilman, the author of the classic novella *The Yellow Wallpaper*, was advised by a famous neurasthenia doctor to 'live as domestic a life as possible. Have your child with you all the time [...]. Lie down an hour after each meal. Have but two hours' intellectual life a day. And never touch pen, brush or pencil as long as you live'.

For others, vigorous exercise was the ticket, alongside dietary changes (sherry, port, plenty of milk), daily massage, electrical stimulation treatment, and climatotherapy (a change of surroundings) – ideally on an ocean cruise or a trip to Atlantic City for its sea air and ocean baths, as recommended in the *Journal of the American Medical Association* (*JAMA*) in February 1899:

> Hot and cold salt-water baths can be obtained all the year, but must not be taken without direction. The average case does best by taking the proper bath every second day, two and one-half hours after breakfast. *Hot* baths are usually detrimental to neurasthenics. Late hours must be prohibited. Every moment possible must be spent in the open air between 10 a.m. and 4 p.m. in the winter, and 9 a.m. and 7 p.m. in summer – not in merry-go-rounds and places of amusement.

Some approaches were more radical: injections of brain tissue from rabbits and sheep, or doses of arsenic, strychnine or opium.

Despite neurasthenia's initial predilection for American society, it soon declared itself in any place where there was social, cultural or political upheaval. Wherever urbanisation and industrialisation began, neurasthenia followed. The translation of Beard's work into German in 1881 saw the condition reach wider attention there, and by 1900 there were at least 500 neurasthenia clinics in Germany. The Austro-German psychiatrist Richard von Krafft-Ebing wrote that 'there is hardly another pathological phenomenon that cuts so deeply into the life of the modern *Culturmensch* as neurasthenia'. In 1897, *L'Hygiène du neurasthénique* (*The Treatment of Neurasthenia*) was published in France, which emphasised the debilitating nature of '*épuisement*' related to 'an incessant and exaggerated function of the nervous system'. It similarly reached mainstream medical attention across much of Europe – there were spas at Karlsbad, Bath, Baden-Baden, Marienbad, Vichy and Teplitz. It emerged in Russia (where putative causes ranged from the 'squandering of sperm' to the wearing of corsets and bustles), and later in China, Japan and Argentina.

In Britain, neurasthenia surfaced in the 1880s, although not everybody set great store by it. The medic Sir Andrew Clark labelled it 'a mob of incoherent symptoms', an understandable reaction to the ever-expanding array of features that appeared in medical texts: weakness of the voice, tenderness of the teeth, yawning, a youthful appearance and a desire for stimulants and narcotics. Nonetheless, the diagnosis made its mark here, across the social divide. In 1886, it appeared at the National Hospital for Neurology and Neurosurgery in Queen Square, London, then known as the National Hospital for the Relief and Cure of the Paralysed and Epileptic, which provided charity treatment for the poor. It accounted for up to a tenth of discharges from the late 1890s to 1930 – similar to the prevalence of brain tumour diagnoses at the time. At the West End Hospital for Diseases of the Nervous System on Welbeck Street, it was the most common diagnosis among all outpatients. A physician to the hospital, Thomas Savill, delivered a series of lectures there in the 1890s, emphasising that the condition was prevalent among the working classes and was 'a disease of clerks'. He believed that nine out of ten patients who presented with 'nervousness' had the condition. In 1904, Seymour J. Sharkey chose neurasthenia and hysteria as the topics of his first address as chair of the Neurological Society of the United Kingdom. He believed that degeneration of nerve cells was the signature of neurasthenia, speaking in detail about experiments on the nervous systems of pigeons and bees, before concluding that 'neurasthenia is one of the most seriously incapacitating conditions'.

Neurasthenia spoke not only to anxieties around social change, it also spoke to national identity. It might not have created that identity, but it certainly could reflect and champion it. Beard had termed neurasthenia 'American nervousness' and viewed it as 'the product of American civilization'. William James referred to it as 'Americanitis'. *McClure's Magazine* called it 'the national disease of America'. The afflicted were 'brain workers', usually men of the 'desk, the pulpit and [...] the counting room', the 'better sort', the 'in-door classes' (the diagnosis later declared itself in manual labourers, but this was not the thrust of Beard's original vision). It was the mark of advanced evolution, of industriousness and ingenuity, of refinement and cerebral sophistication. In the preface to his book *American Nervousness*, Beard's nationalism reaches extraordinary heights: 'All this is modern, and originally American; and no age, no country, and no form of civilization, not Greece, nor Rome, nor Spain, nor the Netherlands, in the days of their glory, possessed such maladies.'

Neurasthenia not only defined America, it elevated it too. The nation's careful study of the condition, Beard wrote, would 'make Europe follow us, instead of our following Europe [...]. Long enough this babyland of science has fed on the crumbs that fall from Germany's table.' Any appearance of the condition in Europe would only symbolise the Americanisation of those lands, an invasion of sorts, albeit a nervous one.

In truth, in Beard's original thesis at least, neurasthenia only defined a certain sort of American. His patients were predominantly Anglo-Saxon middle and upper-class professionals with 'fine, soft hair, delicate skin [and] nicely chiselled features'. Dr J. S. Greene, writing in the *Boston Medical and Surgical Journal* in 1883, believed that 'the Anglo-Saxon race in America, being foremost in development' was 'therefore first to experience the limitations of human capacity'.

Ominously, the Philadelphia physician Charles Burr wrote that neurasthenia could occur in 'half-breeds', but solely in response to 'the struggle of the best specimens of an inferior race to attain the plane of a superior'. Perhaps only a certain sort of person could have neurasthenia, and therefore be considered a choice American specimen.

A narrative centred on national identity emerged in Britain too; not from how neurasthenia affected the British in Britain, but how it afflicted the British abroad. The condition had been diagnosed in Americans stationed in the Philippines in the late nineteenth century, but it became especially prevalent in the British. 'Tropical neurasthenia' typically affected white British men in colonial outposts who exhibited 'an ennui or loss of edge' brought about by the strains of tropical life – its constellation of symptoms paralleled those of the non-tropical form. A series of estimates between 1910 and 1935 consistently named it as one of the leading causes for colonial staff to be repatriated back to

Britain. Invaliding rates from neurasthenia were treble those for men in government service at home.

The condition acquired a distinct regional flavour. Serjeant Surgeon Sir Richard Havelock Charles, in his address to the Royal Society of Tropical Medicine and Hygiene in 1913, reported that during his practice in India he had heard local colleagues say, 'Oh! such and such an [*sic*] one ought to go [back] to Europe for a bit – he has got, or is getting, Punjab head.'

'Punjab head', it transpired, was the term for tropical neurasthenia, which Charles went on to describe more comprehensively:

> An officer, otherwise in every way a good fellow, had become short tempered; forgetful of names; troubled with sleeplessness; given to feel his work too much for him; disinclined to take responsibility; given to make molehills into mountains; procrastinating; susceptible on slight exertion, mental or physical, to fatigue; and with a loss of all powers of concentration. In fact an irritable man, more or less unequal to his work, though otherwise fairly fit.

Audience members enthusiastically told Sir Charles of their encounters with 'Bengal head' and 'Burmese head' in their own colonial staff. Dr Andrew Balfour volunteered his encounter with 'Sudan head', a 'marked disinclination to stoop and look for things near the ground level', which he attributed to laziness: 'So much is this the case that, in Khartoum, we avoided as far as possible having floor cupboards, or placing things in positions which necessitated a stooping posture when looking for them or using them.'

While non-tropical neurasthenia developed in response to urbanisation and industrialisation, tropical neurasthenia was the price paid by decent colonial men dispatched from civilisation for the sake of King and Country. Robert van Someren, retired from the Colonial Service, wrote to the *BMJ* in 1926 to highlight the situation in Uganda. Europeans there, he believed, developed neurasthenia because of 'the unavoidable monotony of life in remote stations, isolated and without any of the great amenities of life; this aggravated by indifferent food, tough African chicken or goat, rendered almost unpalatable by the well meaning intentions of a native cook'. This resulted in ruined digestion, starved nerves and hostility for the foreigner posted there: 'He lacks self-control, everything irritates, and the irascible temper induced easily accounts for such outbursts as one has seen.'

A well-intentioned native cook could seemingly be deemed responsible for their employer's verbal or physical violence. Similar symptoms in the locals might have invited a diagnosis of lunacy, but the diagnosis of tropical neurasthenia conveniently bestowed on colonials a socially tolerable excuse for poor behaviour or for leaving their post – they could be repatriated as invalids rather than as failures or criminals. Sometimes, perhaps, simple exhaustion, melancholy or homesickness lay behind their symptoms. But occasionally and more ominously, a diagnosis of tropical neurasthenia was employed to justify 'sudden acts of violence' and 'acts of criminal folly'. At worst, an outbreak of colonial nerves abdicated aggressors from criminal responsibility.

Either way, a diagnosis of tropical neurasthenia could shield a proud British colonial identity. At an individual level, it spoke to the industrious and refined colonial who endured an oppressively humid climate, becoming neurasthenic only though his over-commitment to labour, through the immense mental strain expended on bettering a nation that called upon his intellect. Tellingly, it was the mark of the colonial officer or missionary but not of the average traveller. The British physician Morden Carthew, advisor to the Thai Department of Health, wrote at the time of a type of traveller called 'the Beachcomber': 'This type is composed of men, usually of the lower classes, of weak moral and mental character and of little will power. He will live a contented life with natives, often adopting their customs. He will seldom develop neurasthenic symptoms.'

At a collective level, maintaining the reputation of the British civil service was paramount to preserving the standing of a nation, as described by one author in 1915: 'The ability, the energy, the industry, and the probity of the British race naturally and obviously have their reflex in the British Civil Service.' Tropical neurasthenia could keep that reputation intact.

As for what to do when an unfortunate sufferer was repatriated, Sir Charles insisted that a replacement be dispatched as soon as possible: 'For a white race to preserve its purity and predominance in a tropical climate, and to keep that vigour, intelligence, and physique which are its characteristics, fresh waves of immigration are essential to make up for the wear and tear due to climatic influences.'

Tropical neurasthenia allowed the colonial officer to be returned home with honour. It also enabled his replacement to be dispatched, so that the nation's dignity could be seen to prevail.

Neurasthenia had been leveraged to showcase individual and national identity: when it could no longer serve this purpose, it began to come unstuck. Those with the condition were increasingly maligned. In 1905, the neuropsychiatrist Smith Ely Jelliffe issued his damning verdict: 'Laziness, indifference, weakness of mind and supersensitiveness characterize them all'. A contemporary of his labelled neurasthenia episodes as 'lapses from productiveness' that 'secure periodic vacations [...] a long rest at some health resort, through an opportune breakdown'. This was hardly the vision Beard had of the idealised modern American or a condition that could be championed as 'the product of American civilization'.

The decline of neurasthenia as a prestigious diagnosis paralleled the rise of eugenics, a term coined by the British scientist Sir Francis Galton, who in his 1883 book *Inquiries into Human Faculty and its Development* described the 'capacity of labour' as 'an attribute of the higher race'. Neurasthenics clearly fell short of this ideal.

By the early twentieth century, eugenic discussions of heredity and degeneracy were re-evaluating the signatures of a favourable stock. In 1913, the British psychiatrist Sir Frederick Mott told the Royal Society of Medicine that neurasthenia might be 'the starting-point of an unstable nervous condition in a stock which in successive generations may intensify under a continuance of an unfavourable environment'. He had a solution: 'Seeing that "like tends to beget like" it will be a good thing for the race when those who are judged to be unfit for social privileges are registered and segregated in early life.'

It's worth placing these opinions alongside the mainstream appeal of eugenics at the time. In 1919, Winston Churchill despaired of the rising number of the 'feeble-minded', which 'constitutes a national and race danger which it is impossible to exaggerate'. He advocated their sterilisation and segregation, 'so that their curse died with them and was not transmitted to future generations'. Four years earlier, Virginia Woolf, after encountering 'a long line of imbeciles on a walk', wrote that 'everyone in that long line was a miserable ineffective shuffling idiotic creature, with no forehead or no chin and an imbecile grin, or a wild, suspicious stare. It was perfectly horrible. They should certainly be killed'. In 1920, Marie Stopes expressed alarm that 'society allows the diseased, the racially negligent, the thriftless, the careless, the feeble-minded, the very lowest and worst members of the community, to produce innumerable tens of thousands of stunted, warped, and inferior infants'.

In Germany at around the same time, neurasthenia had become intimately associated with *erbliche Belastung* ('hereditary burden'). Following the collapse of the Wilhelmine empire in 1918, the neurologist Wilhelm Erb wrote:

> We have to envisage a complete downfall! And this is mainly due to the particular moral comportment of our so-called people, in all its degeneration, laziness, abstinence from work and its craving for pleasure – with all its consequences for the privation of coal, nutrition, and the state order of the Reich.

Erb was not some fringe practitioner. He was the honorary president of the Gesellschaft deutscher Nervenärzte (Society of German Neurologists), and mentored some of the country's best-known scientists and doctors, who drove forward his teachings long after his death in 1921. During the eugenics drive for forced sterilisations in Nazi Germany, it was neurologists and psychiatrists who worked to distinguish between hereditary and acquired disorders, delivered lectures on genetics to SA and SS officials, and served as expert witnesses in Hereditary Health Courts, which selected the patients who would have to undergo forced sterilisation.

Neurasthenia was later parsed in various directions. For the most part, it was relabelled or reconstructed into neuroses such as hysteria, hypochondriasis, maladjustment and compulsivity. At Queen Square, where it was similarly recategorised into the 'psychoneuroses' in 1932, it disappeared entirely after 1941. Cultural anxieties about self and society still existed, but neurasthenia no longer seemed to quite fit.

In other parts of the world, the diagnosis persisted for longer. In China in the 1950s, some clinics reported the condition in up to

90% of their patients; this plague was, according to the psychiatrist Tsung-yi Lin, the result of workers, especially intellectuals, 'laboring under [...] political exhortation and suffering from extreme material, physical, and psychological hardships without any means of venting their frustration or political views' during the Great Leap Forward (1958–62). Sufferers were prescribed sedatives or subjected to re-education therapy to develop 'correct ideas and attitudes to work and socialist life, especially in fostering the proper relationship of the self to the society, the Communist Party, and the nation'. As late as 1982, a study found that 59% of patients with neuroses carried a diagnosis of neurasthenia. In Japan, neurasthenia was for decades seen as a threat to the nation's military – among soldiers, it was attributed to masturbation and 'sexual immorality' – national stability and the social order. A 1992 survey that questioned 166 Japanese psychiatrists found that 70% refused to disclose a diagnosis of schizophrenia to their patients, with 20% opting for a 'euphemistic' substitute diagnosis – neurasthenia accounted for a third of these, even though most psychiatrists were privately reluctant to accept neurasthenia as a diagnosis. Instead, they drew on the term to decrease stigma and spare the feelings of patients and their families.

Its ghost may still linger in the west too. One contemporary diagnostic label is also marked by a constellation of seemingly inexplicable and difficult-to-link symptoms – with debilitating fatigue at its core – and the absence of a definitive confirmatory test: that diagnosis is chronic fatigue syndrome (CFS). Up to 97% of patients with CFS in one study also met criteria for neurasthenia, but that's not to say that CFS is synonymous with neurasthenia. More recently, parallels have been drawn between burnout and neurasthenia – burnout provides a similar picture of physical and mental exhaustion, and both conditions are attributed to a strong commitment – perhaps over-commitment – to work, are both characterised by an assemblage of physical symptoms such as headaches, insomnia and stomach problems, and share a context of novel technologies that force us to be always 'connected'; and there is even a high prevalence of them in physicians (as seemed to be the case with neurasthenia).

In the construction and application of these nineteenth-century diagnoses, the hegemony of the medical establishment was fully realised. Despite their flaws and fallacies, spermatorrhea, status lymphaticus and neurasthenia not only reflected the concerns of their age but also afforded medicine power and privilege, authority and agency. That legacy remains, and has ultimately informed all that followed. The diagnosis of spermatorrhea, in particular, set the scene for the wholesale medicalisation of sexual preoccupations, and the medical establishment's foray into the pathologisation of sexual deviancy. In the next chapter, I will meet Jeremy and Sarah, whose 'diagnoses' of homosexuality stemmed from that process. They have both, against all the odds, lived to tell the tale.

The Deviancy Diagnosis

Lynfield Mount Hospital
Heights Lane
Bradford BD9 6DP

1 June 1972

Dr R Brogden
130 Skipton Road
Keighley

Dear Ruth

Re Jeremy Gavins
68 Devonshire Street, Keighley

[...] This boy [...] has homosexual desires and fantasies. [...]
When one goes into his sexuality in greater detail, there is little
doubt that he has both heterosexual and homosexual fantasies
associated with masturbation, but the homosexual tend to be
dominant. He has masturbatory guilt both related to his religion
and external to his religion. [...] What we should do at this
stage is to try and avert him to his homosexual fantasies by
aversion techniques and by operant conditioning encourage his
heterosexual desires. This our Clinical Psychologist will undertake

and I will continue to see the boy with a view to trying to help
him psychotherapeutically as far as his personality disorder is
concerned.
Yours sincerely,
[signed]
[p.p.] H. B. Milne
Consultant Psychiatrist

A priest had walked Jeremy to his appointment with Hugo Milne
at Lynfield Mount Hospital. They had left unnoticed by the back
gate of Jeremy's school, walked up Leylands Lane, across Toller Lane,
then to the end of Duchy Drive and across to the hospital. It took
fifteen minutes. They didn't talk. Jeremy was eighteen years old.

Six days later, Jeremy returned to the hospital. A man in a white
coat told him to strip, then to put on a dressing gown and slippers.
The slippers were too big; they made a 'flip-flop' noise as he was
led to a treatment room. There, he had to sit in a wooden chair
that had a straight back and arms. His wrists were fastened down
with leather straps. A grey band was attached to his right forearm,
and the band's electric wires were connected to a box on a table
in front of him. The man in the white coat opened Jeremy's gown
to see if he was aroused. He was not.

The lights were turned down.

He was shown pictures of men and women, most of them
naked. Electric shocks accompanied each picture of a naked
man, but not the pictures of the women. With each jolt, Jeremy's
arm would contort, his body would spasm. He was there for an
hour and twenty minutes. More sessions each week, for months.
Those electric shocks pulsed through his body for years; or at least
seemed to.

Jeremy's behaviour was deemed deviant by religious institutions,
and later called 'diseased' by medical ones. In its characterisation

of homosexuality as sinful, the religious establishment secured the right to decide what was aberrant and what was not. The medical establishment followed in its footsteps; but when it labelled homosexuality as a psychiatric diagnosis, it supposedly did this so that patients could be helped and healed, rather than castigated and criminalised. Jeremy's story shows us how a diagnostic label defined the treatment he was subjected to; and how, even now, the religious establishment has never really stepped away at all.

Jeremy was fourteen years old when he fell in love with a boy called Stephen. 'If you want to know what he looked like,' Jeremy tells me, 'he looked like the singer Donovan, a younger version. Black curly hair, a nice kissable nose as well. About the same height as me, but he was slim. I was the rough, chunky rugby-playing type and he was arty, more delicate.'

They were friends to begin with, but two years later Jeremy told him that 'I think you are the most beautiful boy in the world. I love you.' Stephen felt the same way.

Jeremy's parents would not have approved. 'At St Bede's, a Catholic grammar school, there were statues, but it were just as bad at home, because my parents were Catholic. Very, very, very Catholic.'

The family lived in Keighley, a former mill town eleven miles north-west of Bradford, along the Worth near its confluence with the Aire. A restored steam line, featured in *The Railway Children*, runs from there to Haworth, home of the Brontës, and Oxenhope. Bert and Betty saw their son as the cassock-wearing 'good little altar boy'. Jeremy had experimented with boys from the age of eleven, first with Martin, in an old barn in some fields behind a park. Martin was good-looking too. 'George Clooney at the age of eleven. He had a Yorkshire sense of humour.' What's a Yorkshire sense of humour, I ask? 'It's just odd, taking the piss out of anything.' Later, Jeremy's experimentation with other young boys moved elsewhere – in the woods, once in the public toilets, at scout camp. Above all, in secret.

Now aged sixty-seven, Jeremy lives in Ulverston, some 70 miles from his childhood home. His rescue dog Timmy ('part collie, part fox') sits at his feet. Next to the wood burner on its stone hearth are a pile of notebooks, filled with details of the drystone walls he has built for decades. He still has the build of a rugby player. On his black T-shirt are Snoopy and Peanuts: 'In a world where you can be anything, be kind.'

There's not much hair on the top of his head, but his white beard makes up for that. 'Timmy, he sits on me knee and he licks me face all over, and my beard. If I have something with gravy for me tea, he likes that.'

Stephen became the love of Jeremy's life. He still is, or at least the memory of him is. They spent as much time as they could with one another at school. They went to a gay pub once, but it was too much of a risk to be seen together. They sang Diana Ross songs. Stephen called him 'Jeremy the Sugar Puffs Bear'. What did you call him? 'Stephen, just Stephen.'

As their A-levels approached, it became clear they would be going to different universities in different towns, a devastating realisation for Jeremy. A teacher found him collapsed and crying alone in the corridor. 'What's wrong?' Answering that question truthfully was the gravest mistake he has ever made, says Jeremy. He explained he was in love, then admitted it was with Stephen. The teacher, a priest, listened carefully for a while. Then he told Jeremy he was abnormal, sick and sinful. He was brought to the headmaster, Monsignor Sweeney. Homosexuality was a terrible affliction, said the monsignor. He was much shorter than Jeremy, but in that moment, all-powerful, he seemed a towering presence.

Banned from seeing Stephen again, Jeremy was given two

choices: expulsion before his A-levels (his parents would be told why, and he would miss out on university – his impending escape route from home) or curative treatment during them. 'We can stop you feeling like this, we can heal you of your disease,' said the monsignor. It was hardly a choice at all.

He was sent by the monsignor to his (Catholic) family doctor who, without discussion or hesitation, referred him to a psychiatrist.

The psychiatrist saw him for one consultation before the aversion therapy. 'The initial treatment was carried out by some underling, I don't know, I never found [out] the name, but everything was directed by Hugo Milne.'

The first electric shock sent a stabbing, burning pain piercing through his right forearm. 'It's supposed to hurt,' the man in the white coat said. More shocks followed. When he tried to look away from the pictures, he was told to look back at them.

If the pain got too much, the man in the white coat said, he could avert a shock by flicking the switch in his left hand to bring up a picture of a woman. That was a lie, Jeremy discovered – the switch did not work eighty per cent of the time. These mind games were all part of the treatment.

Back at school, the monsignor warned Jeremy not to tell his parents about his 'illness' or treatment. 'Once you are cured, you won't need to tell them anyway.'

Later, Jeremy discovered the priests had told his parents the truth. They had known about the electric shock therapy all along, and did nothing to stop it.

Psychiatrists at the hospital administered Jeremy's treatment, but priests took him there. I ask Jeremy who bears ultimate responsibility? 'The Catholic Church,' he answers, immediately. 'It didn't occur to me at the time, cos it never does because you are eighteen and you don't know what you're doing, but they took over. They knew what to do. They told me to go and see me GP, and then they asked me if I had got the letter from the loony bin and they walked me up to the loony bin. They could have sent for a nurse to take me or they could have sent me in a taxi, or I could have walked up, but to be actually walked up there by the school … they knew all about it.'

But he also knows that the treatment he received was sanctioned by a psychiatric diagnosis. Homosexuality had officially been classified a mental disorder. The 1948 edition of the WHO's diagnostic manual had labelled homosexuality as aberrant, including it in its category of 'sexual deviation' alongside exhibitionism, fetishism, pathologic sexuality and sadism. In the 1975 edition, 'sexual deviation' was defined as sexual activity 'directed primarily towards people not of the opposite sex, or towards sexual acts not associated with coitus normally, or towards coitus performed under abnormal circumstances'. The roots of medical diagnosis are deeply entangled with religious ones. 'It's always up to doctors, isn't it?' Jeremy says. 'When it comes to homosexuality, the doctor who is Christian and believes in the Bible more than the Hippocratic Oath [is] acting as a Christian, not as a medical person. What they should have said is, "What we should do with this boy is talk to him and figure out what's going on in his head", rather than immediately sending me off down that road so quick.'

When he came out to his parents some years later, his mother suggested it was a phase. His father told Jeremy he had robbed the word 'gay' of its 'lovely' meaning for him. He spoke of the Bible, he spoke of sin, he spoke of shame and disgust and humiliation, then he left the room.

Who was responsible for deciding that Jeremy's love for Stephen was abnormal, that he – then a teenager – deserved to be strapped to a wooden chair and brutalised with electric shocks? And how did these judgements come to pass?

★

In the eighteenth and nineteenth centuries, as the Church's authority in the west diminished – and the power of the medical establishment grew – the categories of demonic possession, drunkenness and sodomy were redesignated insanity, alcoholism and homosexuality. Deviancy, as Howard Becker wrote in 1963, 'is not a quality that lies in behavior itself, but in the interaction between the person who commits an act and those who respond to it'.

And yet the term of homosexuality was originally coined as a call to reform, by the Hungarian journalist Károly Mária Kertbeny in 1869. His manifesto criticised Prussian laws that criminalised same-sex relations between men, arguing that '*Homosexualität*' was a normal, immutable variation, and could never 'be suppressed even by the most brutal persecutions'. But the term was soon appropriated by doctors, including the German psychiatrist Richard von Krafft-Ebing. In his influential 1886 book, *Psychopathia Sexualis*, he labelled '*die konträre Sexualempfindung*' ('the contrary sexual instinct') as a form of 'degeneracy' to rank alongside sadism and masochism.

Over the course of the nineteenth century, the rest of the medical establishment had secured a commanding position thanks to an improved understanding of infectious diseases like yellow fever, smallpox, typhus and cholera, but the rising discipline of psychiatry was broadly perceived to offer social cures rather than scientific ones. Now, psychiatrists had an opportunity to elevate the status of the discipline through becoming the gatekeepers of deviancy.

The diagnostic label of homosexuality allowed psychiatrists to become the purveyors of moral concerns, delineating rigidly what was pathological and what wasn't, what violated the constructed boundaries of normality or did not, what was sexually aberrant and what was not. As the sociologist Eliot Freidson wrote in 1972,

'Where illness is the ubiquitous label for deviance in an age, the profession that is custodian of the label is ascendant.'

In subsequent decades, the WHO's decision to classify homosexuality as a disorder was influential in embedding it into medical practice. The American Psychiatric Association (APA) likewise included homosexuality in the first edition of its classification manual – the 1952 *Diagnostic and Statistical Manual of Mental Disorders* (DSM). In the DSM, 'sexual deviations' were categorised as 'sociopathic personality disturbances'. This was the broad international context, but there were also proceedings closer to home that would influence the treatment of Jeremy and others who were handed the same diagnosis.

Among the documents held in the archive of the BMA are the records of a meeting scheduled for Monday, 6 December 1954. The record announces that T. H. Blench (Manchester), T. C. N. Gibbens (Kingswood, Surrey), R. G. Gibson (Winchester), Professor J. Glaister (Glasgow) and six other members of the association met for the first in a series of discussions. Drawn from psychiatry, venereology, general practice and forensic medicine, they represented one of a number of groups, including clergy and prominent gay men, who had been asked to give evidence to the Wolfenden Committee, established by the Conservative government in 1954 to conduct an inquiry into the legality of homosexuality and prostitution. This innocuous-looking collection of papers from the BMA is evidence of a medical establishment fearful that homosexuality would tear the social fabric of the nation.

The BMA experts chose to focus on male homosexuality – its 'nature and causes [...] control and cure' – since 'female homosexuality has never presented a serious social problem'. An expert was summoned to comment on genetic and environmental 'variations in sexual polarity'. Preliminary evidence was presented of physical and behavioural characteristics allegedly unique to homosexual men and present in up to half of those studied: 'subnormal growth of facial and public hair, span of outstretched arms greater than height, voice high in excitement, artistic temperament and excessive sensitivity, and inadequacy at games and running'. Various subtypes were proposed: 'well-compensated homosexuals of good character, often greatly helped by psychotherapy'; 'seriously damaged personalities, sometimes intensely lonely, shy, and inadequate persons whose only affectionate or social contact may be in fleeting lavatory offences or minor play with children'; individuals who were 'of a very effeminate and essentially narcissistic make-up who like to be admired and feather their nest'; as well as 'antisocial and often aggressive characters, with a mixture of other perversions, especially fetishism and sadomasochism, with homosexuality'.

Medical intervention was not needed for all, the committee decided; sometimes moral encouragement would do. Electro-convulsive therapy and drug treatment were useful 'for the accompanying mental illness rather than for the homosexual con-dition itself'. Oestrogens could 'produce cessation or diminution of sexual desire in most subjects'.

There were some mild attempts at conciliation – the committee decided it was 'inadequate for society to condemn the conduct of homosexuals', for instance – but these were soon undone by their conclusions:

> Some [male] homosexuals appear to be incorrigible
> offenders, often inveterate and degenerate sodomists and
> debauchers of youth. Even after repeated conviction,
> imprisonment, and treatment they still persist in their
> conduct, and they should be dealt with in the same
> way as mentally deranged offenders. In the BMA's

recommendations to the Royal Commission on the
Law relating to Mental Disease and Deficiency the
establishment of institutions for psychopathic patients
on the lines of a colony under disciplinary control and
with psychiatric advice and treatment is suggested. Some
incorrigible offenders might be found to be psychopaths
who could best be treated in such institutions.

The publication of the committee's memorandum in the *BMJ*
of December 1955 was well received: 'a masterly report which
clarifies the whole subject', wrote Robert Browne of Birmingham
B20, in his letter to the editor. 'The guardians of the nation's health
may well be concerned with the moral climate of the country and
be grateful for this clear and courageous lead.' A report 'wide in
its conception', pronounced Denis Ellison Nash of London W1,
encouraging the association to continue to 'give a lead in any
moral issue which in the end may affect the spiritual and thus the
mental and physical well-being of the community'.

There was the occasional note of dissent. S. L. Sherwood of
London W14 wrote that the report had caused him a great deal
of apprehension: 'As I remember it, the Hippocratic Oath charges
us with alleviating suffering and at all times loyalty to our patients
[...]. Our oath says nothing about legislation, administration, or
morals – they are, in our tradition, not our business except that
part of conduct which concerns our own.'

It's clear, to my mind, that Sherwood's voice was utterly
drowned out by those who believed the morals of the nation were
the purview of the medical establishment, as evidenced by the
tone of the committee's report:

At the present time there is no lack of stimulation to
the sexual appetite. Suggestive advertisements abound,

provocative articles and illustrations appear in the
newspapers; magazines and cheap novels with lurid
covers frequently provide suggestive reading matter, and
the erotic nature of many films and stage shows is but
thinly veiled.

This chilling intrusion of the medical establishment into the moral
sphere validated the heinous medical interventions that Jeremy
and others faced. One doctor who carried out aversion therapy in
Bristol wrote that he had been spurred on by the 1955 BMA report
that had 'laid stress on the need for research into the treatment of
homosexuals'. This is the power of bestowing a behaviour with a
diagnostic label: it advocates or mandates control and cure.

The Wolfenden Committee resolutely refused, however, to
see homosexuality in pathological terms: 'Homosexuality cannot
legitimately be regarded as a disease, because in many cases it is the
only symptom and is compatible with full mental health in other
respects.' The committee concluded in 1957 that 'homosexual
behaviour between consenting adults in private should no longer
be considered a criminal offence', deeming the age of consent to
be twenty-one (the heterosexual age of consent at the time was
sixteen in England, Scotland and Wales, and seventeen in Northern
Ireland). This recommendation that male homosexuality should
be partly decriminalised was not realised until the Sexual Offences
Act 1967 was passed in England and Wales. Similar legislation
followed for Scotland in 1980 and Northern Ireland in 1982.

Critically, this relatively progressive thinking – at least in so far
as it rejected the claim that 'homosexuality' is a disease – was not
echoed within the international medical establishment. The WHO
continued to include homosexuality in its *International Statistical
Classification of Diseases and Related Health Problems* (ICD). The APA
persisted in listing it in the DSM too: by the time of the DSM's second

edition, the 1968 DSM–II, eight sexual deviations were included, all clearly demarcated as mental disorders: homosexuality, fetishism, paedophilia, transvestism, exhibitionism, voyeurism, sadism and masochism. These inclusions jarred against the growing influence of Alfred Kinsey, whose publications *Sexual Behavior in the Human Male* (1948) and *Sexual Behavior in the Human Female* (1953) spoke to a range of sexual behaviours in the general population that were more common than the diagnostic designation of deviancy might suggest. But as the psychotherapist Gary Greenberg has written of the DSM, 'it is as important to psychiatrists as the Constitution is to the US government or the Bible is to Christians'. And in the aftermath of the BMA's report, and despite the eventual change in the law, 'therapies' for the diagnosis of homosexuality continued to be provided in the UK – as Jeremy would discover in the early 1970s, with each trip to Lynfield Mount Hospital. The priests may have walked him up there, but it was decisions made further afield that had sealed his fate.

Discriminatory attitudes to homosexuality prevailed well in advance of the diagnostic classifications in the DSM and ICD, and the conclusions of the BMA experts. Social, religious, political and legal forces conspired to judge same-sex behaviours long before those medical opinions emerged. Although the death penalty for acts of sodomy was abolished in 1861 in England, Wales and Ireland, they were still punishable by imprisonment, with a minimum ten-year sentence. The Criminal Law Amendment Act 1885 outlawed any male homosexual act, even in private (Oscar Wilde fell foul of this in 1895 and was sentenced to two years of hard labour). Sodomy remained a capital offence in Scotland until 1889.

In 1920s Germany, researchers transplanted testicles from heterosexual donors to homosexual recipients to drive 'heterosexual function' in the latter group. Before long, sterilisation was being used as a tool of eugenic control: those suspected of homosexual offences were regularly subjected to the same castration techniques as those found guilty of child sexual abuse, under the 1933 Law Against Habitual Criminals and Sex Offenders. In 1941, the death penalty was introduced for men in the police and SS convicted of homosexual offences.

Just over a decade later, the British mathematician and code-breaker Alan Turing underwent chemical castration after being convicted of gross indecency over his relationship with another man. Ordered to take oestrogen to reduce his sex drive, he later took his own life.

In the years leading up to the publication of the DSM, being suspected by the FBI of homosexuality resulted in 1,700 people being denied employment between January 1947 and August 1950, while 4,380 people were discharged from the military for homosexuality over the same period. A senate inquiry at the time stated that homosexuals should not be employed by the government because of a propensity for criminal and immoral behaviour, a lack of emotional stability ('indulgence in acts of sex perversion weakens the moral fibre'), a 'tendency to gather other perverts' around them and a heightened security risk ('the pervert is easy prey to the blackmailer').

But enshrining homosexuality within medical classification systems, especially in an environment where same-sex attraction already faced opprobrium, validated decisions far beyond the consensus meetings and conferences where doctors gathered. Take the DSM's early classification of homosexuality as a 'sociopathic personality disturbance': this designation coincided in the US with the Immigration and Nationality Act 1952, which stated that the list of those who 'shall be excluded from admission into the United States' included 'aliens afflicted with psychopathic personality'. This legislation was drawn upon some years later in a US Supreme Court case which led to the deportation of the Canadian national Clive Boutilier on the grounds of homosexuality.

Meanwhile, Jeremy and others discovered that a medical diagnosis meant that they were seemingly judged just as harshly within hospital walls as outside them. Instead of therapy, they were subjected to torment. It is the implications of this diagnostic labelling with regard to treatment that I explore next.

Those who defined homosexuality as a perversion often proclaimed to do so in the interest of compassion and in the spirit of reformation (of law and public opinion). A medical model, they argued, had the power to redefine same-sex attraction as a form of sickness instead of a sin or criminal offence, and so the perceived deviant should be freed from blame and steered towards a cure rather than a prison sentence. But this thesis – that medicalising something, conferring on it a diagnostic label, inevitably brings healing – is deeply flawed.

A diagnosis that labelled a behaviour as aberrant could justify treatments, sometimes appalling ones, in the name of scientific understanding and medical advancement. Because homosexuality was viewed specifically as a deviant behaviour, patients were subjected to the same treatments as other conditions of perceived deviancy, including alcoholism and drug addiction. The BMA committee report of 1955 proposed experimental treatment centres, 'similar in function to "Alcoholics Anonymous"', where 'inmates' should follow a routine of work, exercise and study, with strict discipline and supervision: 'In no case would individuals be discharged until there was clear evidence of their sound reformation.'

Crucially, an official diagnosis of homosexuality awarded agency to those who diagnosed it, gifting them an authority that is epitomised by the story of Luchia Fitzgerald, who ran away from

Ireland after her family discovered she was gay and threatened to send her to an asylum. She recalled a conversation between her psychiatrist and probation officer in the late 1950s or early 1960s:

> They were discussing how they could put it right and he made some suggestions of a part of my brain not being developed right and that really ... the only way forward was to have surgery ... I was thinking to myself maybe these people are right because they're professionals, they know what they're doing ... I thought maybe if I was heterosexual, I could go home, settle down and be like everybody else. So, I thought, well, if these people can cure me, I'm going to let them.

She changed her mind after a conversation with a friend at the pub, and narrowly evaded potential lifelong disability or perhaps even death.

At the time, a technique called aversion therapy was used across the UK to recondition sexual behaviours, and was mainly inflicted on men.* Like Jeremy, they were subjected to electric shocks, or injected with drugs that induced nausea and vomiting as they viewed erotic images of people of the same sex. These men, claimed the psychiatrists and psychologists who conducted this treatment, would be turned away from their homosexuality – a behaviour that would now be inextricably connected in their minds with emotional trauma and physical pain. Extensive use

---

* Anecdotal evidence shows that women were also subjected to aversion therapy, although less frequently than men. The true numbers are unknown: they were less likely to be subjected to these treatments as punishment for a criminal offence (female same-sex attraction was not criminalised), and the absence of criminalisation means that we do not have figures for how many women underwent treatment.

of aversion therapy for homosexuality was first made in Prague in the 1950s by the psychiatrist and sexologist Kurt Freund, whose initial enthusiasm for the technique was tempered by his later findings, when he discovered that the 'motivation' of those patients whom he followed up on for several years was 'still almost exclusively homosexual'. He ended up campaigning to repeal anti-homosexual laws in Czechoslovakia.

But Freund's eventual ambivalence regarding the effectiveness of aversion therapy did not hamper its importation into the UK. The most influential proponent of his work was Hans Eysenck at the Institute of Psychiatry at King's College London, who at the time of his death was the third most cited psychologist of all time after Sigmund Freud and Jean Piaget. Eysenck translated Freund's work, making it known to a British audience. He even hosted Freund at his department at the Maudsley Hospital in London, alongside a score of psychiatrists and psychologists who would go on to practise the techniques they learnt there.

An understanding of diagnosis goes hand in hand with an understanding of the dominant figures in a profession, those who educate and inspire the next generation. Recently, the Royal College of Psychiatrists (RCPsych) gathered some mental health specialists who practised at psychiatric hospitals in the 1960s. Reflecting on their experiences back then, two psychiatrists, Harry Zeitlin and Peter Tyrer, gave this account (slightly abridged):

> Zeitlin: [...] Eysenck had a huge influence.
> Tyrer: But Eysenck never treated a patient. Let's
> remember that.
> Zeitlin: But he treated us. I listened to him lecturing
> every week, all the time. [...]
> Tyrer: [...] In the sixties when someone very important
> made a statement or made an observation about a

clinical problem, that [...] was regarded as evidence. So, when people like Sargant [a psychiatrist] and Eysenck and everybody else made these statements, they were our figures of authority and we agreed with their judgments.

It was only after Eysenck's death in 1997 that long-standing concerns about scientific fraud and misconduct in his work on personality and behaviour reached the mainstream. In 2019, King's itself concluded that the results of many of Eysenck's studies were 'unsafe', and numerous journals have since retracted his papers.

One early British case report of aversion therapy citing Eysenck's work came from a young Bristol psychiatrist called Basil James, in 1962. James described the scientific approach he used in 'a 40-year-old 100% homosexual': the patient was given an injection every two hours to induce nausea; whenever the man experienced nausea 'a strong light was shone on a large piece of card on which were pasted several photographs of nude or near-nude men'. He was asked to select the man he found most attractive and then fantasise about his current male partner.

> Thereafter a tape was played twice over every two hours during the period of nausea [...] the adverse effect [of his homosexual experiences] and its consequent social repercussions was then described in slow and graphic terms ending with words such as 'sickening', 'nauseating' etc., followed by the noise of one vomiting.

James called the treatment a resounding success. Not only had the man apparently become entirely heterosexual after a week of treatment, he had also become a prolific writer: 'In the 20 weeks since his treatment he has written several short stories, some of which have been accepted by publishers, and has completed a full-length novel.'

His article in the *BMJ* invited some criticism for its brief follow up of only a single case, but there were several favourable responses, including one from a Lincolnshire doctor who wrote that James's work would 'have brought hope to some of the unhappy million homosexuals in this country', and from another doctor who wrote that 'the treatment of homosexuality [...] is usually disappointing and success of even one case is, therefore, an outstanding achievement [...]. Any innovation in the treatment giving successful results is worthy of publication if only in the hope of encouraging others to make further attempts to establish its value.'

This case report and others that documented aversion therapy at the time reached the national press – the *Observer* published an article titled 'How doctor cured a homosexual' and the *Sunday Pictorial's* piece was headlined '"Twilight" men can be cured'. However, another story that year did not make it into the academic or popular press: 29-year-old army captain Billy Clegg-Hill died during court-ordered aversion therapy using apomorphine – the same drug used by Basil James – at a military hospital at Netley near Southampton. His death certificate stated he died from 'natural causes'; the truth emerged only decades later.

Other psychologists and psychiatrists began to train in these aversion techniques, and although it is difficult to ascertain precisely how many men were subjected to aversion, we do know it was at least several hundred – it was not a fringe practice, even if it was not mainstream. Papers outlining its use were widely published in leading academic journals, with claims that it eliminated homosexual interests and retrained patients 'in the essential social preliminaries of heterosexual behaviour', as researchers from the University of Birmingham wrote in 1970. There were treatment hubs in Glasgow, Surrey, Manchester and Birmingham, as well as individual researchers using the technique in London, Leicester,

Barrow Gurney (near Bristol), Lancashire and Belfast. A treatment unit for homosexuality was established in 1964 at the Crumpsall Hospital in Manchester, as covered by *The Times*, the *Guardian* and the *Scotsman*.

Others who visited or worked in Eysenck's department went on to import the technique into their own subsequent practice. One of these, the psychiatrist Nathaniel McConaghy, was still using aversion therapy with electric shocks in the 1980s at the Prince of Wales Hospital in Randwick, New South Wales, although he admitted that 'some subjects who showed a [degree] of heterosexual orientation before treatment showed a change in the homosexual direction'.

At the Maudsley, the psychiatrist John Bancroft employed an electric shock technique similar to that used on Jeremy. Bancroft's patients were shown 'photographs chosen to produce erotic homosexual fantasies'. He described his methods in a 1969 paper:

> Painful electric shocks were delivered to his arm
> whenever an erection developed up to a certain
> level [usually around 0.6 mm increase in penile
> circumference] [...] further shocks were given at 15
> second intervals unless the erectile response was falling
> or was once again below the threshold level. A minimum
> of 5 shocks was given in any one trial. On the average,
> 12 such trials were given in each session.

Each patient received 30–40 sessions and each session lasted up to 90 minutes. The results, Bancroft admitted, were modest, with 'a reduction in homosexual interest and behaviour [although] homosexuality still predominates over heterosexuality'. He assessed the success of this treatment with a questionnaire he had devised, which asked whether the subject subsequently dated women, found his wife 'sexually interesting' or experienced 'revulsion during homosexual acts'.

According to Bancroft, the most successful treatment was on a 37-year-old zoologist, described as conscientious, highly intelligent and 'of sound personality'. Two and a half years after his 35 sessions, he had maintained a conditioned 'phobic' anxiety to potentially attractive males, experiencing a 'pang of discomfort in the chest when seeing them'. 'Success' came at a high price. After the treatment, the zoologist tried to kill himself when a male friend became engaged to a woman. During a six-month relationship with a woman, 'he had a constant fear of impotence which prevented him from attempting genital contact'.

Bancroft's conclusion was that 'although unpleasant, the treatment has been tolerated well, and in no case can the patient be said to be worse off as a result of it'. And yet, another patient, a 22-year-old, had attempted suicide, a 47-year-old had experienced 'quite severe depression' and a 27-year-old had developed transient psychosis. Others developed high levels of anxiety during treatment and some, he wrote, developed impotence in both homosexual and heterosexual encounters, eventually rejecting relationships entirely.

The presence of homosexuality in respected international diagnostic classifications helped to legitimise medical interventions elsewhere too. Perhaps one of the most extreme examples happened in West Germany, where by 1979 at least 70 men had undergone brain surgery to cure their purported sexual deviancy. Two influential surgeons, Fritz Roeder and Dieter Müller, based their method of 'curing homosexuality' on the findings of animal mating experiments, captured on film by two of their colleagues, Leon Schreiner and Arthur Kling:

'This film which Schreiner and Kling showed […] was a veritable mine of information on human sexual pathology […] the behavior of male cats with lesions of the amygdala region in some respects closely approached that of human perversion. The films convinced us that there was a basis for a therapeutic, [surgical] approach to this problem in man.'

Roeder and Müller began to operate on similar regions of the brain in men with 'homosexual deviation', presenting their results at international conferences. The researchers concluded that their techniques were effective – results were 'in most cases excellent with complete harmonisation of sexual and social behaviour'. It is unknown if any of the men died during or after surgery, although case reports referred to 'reduction in total sex drive', 'dizzy spells', 'ravenous hunger', and a 'tendency to verbal aggression'.

The medical establishment's drive to pathologise same-sex attraction, to pursue cure at any cost, left deep scars.

Jeremy's aversion therapy sessions took place during his A-levels, and because he had a conditional offer from the University of Exeter he asked his teachers if the treatment could be deferred until after the exams. They refused. He failed them all, writing stories instead of numbers in his Maths exam, walking out of others to get drunk at the pub across the road, not even turning up for the rest. He was forced to redo the year at St Bede's and subjected to another six months of aversion therapy. If he missed a session, the priest would find him and drive him there. In later sessions administered by his psychiatrist, the picture slides disappeared. Instead, he was told to imagine himself and Stephen naked. There were electric shocks when he could do this and shocks when he could not. He was made to listen to recordings from his earlier sessions. He was told to forget about Stephen because Stephen hated him. At the end of the year, Jeremy failed his exams again.

By the time he was 25, Jeremy had stepped away from relationships and sex completely. His life was marked by depression and anxiety, by alcohol dependence and agonising chronic pain.

He was haunted then by what, much later, turned out to be a false memory, though for decades he believed it entirely: sometime during those months of aversion therapy as a teenager, he thought he had witnessed the last moments of the boy he loved. The boy with the curly hair and the kissable nose, the boy who got off a bus as a blizzard swirled around them, the boy who slipped as he ran towards Jeremy, the boy who was hit by an oncoming car. The collision became a memory he could not erase. Stephen, and the love they shared and the death he believed he had seen, became, by his own admission, a lifetime's obsession.

From his twenties onwards, Jeremy led a peripatetic life, working in a textile mill early on, then on the railways – shovelling stone and cutting down trees. He built drystone walls here and there, went ice-climbing on the Old Man of Coniston and walked the Langdales in the Lake District. He coppiced woodlands, felled hazel trees to bring in light, he says, to bring in living things, to allow things to live. He dug turf within the ruins of Deer Abbey, the old Cistercian monastery near Aberdeen. He built log bridges in the Fairy Glen near Rosemarkie and at the Birks of Aberfeldy. He built drystone walls at Brodie Castle near Nairn and on the beach on the Orkney island of Rousay. He put up fencing across peat bogs on Hoy in the Shetlands and planted trees on the Isle of Rùm off Skye.

He tried to kill himself many times, getting drunk and passing out in the snow, or standing in the middle of the road, waiting to be hit by a car (he managed a fractured arm but emerged otherwise unscathed, physically at least).

His parents both died in 2015. The last time Jeremy met his father, they did not speak. As he wrote later in his memoir, *Is it About That Boy?*: 'To him I was still the sinful queer boy, and to me, he was the man who represented everything I hated about the Catholic religion.'

To this day, instead of slippers, Jeremy wears old walking boots with laces undone. He cannot wear a watch or a shirt with buttoned cuffs: both remind him of the straps the man in the white coat used to tie him down.

Not all people who underwent this kind of treatment were forced to do so by authority figures, like Jeremy, or as part of a criminal sentence. Medical professionals who truly felt a duty to help gay, lesbian or gender non-conforming people who came to them in need might have rationalised in their minds that doling out even physically and psychologically damaging treatments was better than rejecting their patients entirely. One man admitted to psychiatric hospital for treatment recalled reading a newspaper article about how gay men could be cured and thinking to himself: 'No longer was I an evil pervert. Now I believed I could be viewed as a patient with all the vulnerabilities and sympathy a patient demands.'

Many professionals later insisted they had little choice in the matter. In a 2004 survey, two psychologists who administered aversion therapy spoke of their experiences:

> Here were people coming along who seemed to be
> asking for help, it was against the law, they wanted to
> change their behaviour, that's how it was presented to us.
> You never thought about the morality of what you were
> doing. You were effectively a technician.

And:

> Well, I didn't have much choice. That was a clinical
> placement. I was [the consultant's] first student. Basically,
> the first year I was there, more or less all I ever did was
> shove electricity down homosexual patients.

John Bancroft (whose 1960s research on aversion therapy I mentioned earlier) later went on to lead the Kinsey Institute for Research in Sex, Gender, and Reproduction at Indiana University. In a *New York Times* interview in 1999, he was asked about his past:

> Q. When you were a sex therapist in Great Britain, you did aversion therapy on homosexual patients. Do you regret that now?
>
> A. I don't regret it because I think my motives for doing it were entirely honorable. I just think it was a stage of development in the way we were thinking about it. I am embarrassed about it when people discover it.
>
> Q. Do you fear you damaged your patients?
>
> A. No, not at all.
>
> Q. Or perhaps, wasted their time?
>
> A. Oh, I think I must have wasted many patients' times [*sic*] over the years. Yes, I think it was a fruitless exercise, but it didn't take me very long to realize that.
>
> Q. Do you consider homosexuality a sickness?
>
> A. No. Not at all.
>
> Q. Then why do aversion therapy?
>
> A. Because one was responding to individuals coming along and saying, 'I want to change.' I still respect that request. It's a request that one gets seldom or never, now. The individual who is wanting to deal with his sexual life, I'm there to try to help them sort it out, one way or the other.

But this idea of patients 'volunteering' for treatment was not always accurate, and even those who signed up to treatment, seemingly voluntarily, were not always aware of what lay ahead. Treated with nausea-inducing drugs in 1964, comedian and DJ Peter Price was hospitalised for three days and left 'in a bed smeared with his own vomit and faeces'. In 1996 he told *The Independent* that the treatment at Chester Hospital had destroyed 30 years of his life:

> If I'd known what they were going to do to me, I would
> never have gone in [...] I feel that something was messed
> around in my head. Sometimes I find myself preaching
> to gay people, asking: do you realise what you're doing
> is wrong? But what have I been doing? Having sex with
> men. It's bizarre, like a poison in my mind.

He later saw the psychiatrist who had treated him at a gay club in Manchester.

One perhaps unexpected truth is that some gay activists themselves, doctors included, did not reject the designation of homosexuality as a psychiatric diagnosis; in fact, they supported it. As Jack Drescher – a US psychiatrist and psychoanalyst, and later MD of GALA (Gay and Lesbian Analysts) – has written: 'Some mid-20th century homophile (gay) activist groups accepted psychiatry's illness model as an alternative to societal condemnation of homosexuality's "immorality" and were willing to work with professionals who sought to "treat" and "cure" homosexuality.'

But the creation of a diagnostic label undoubtedly did not just sanction the use of egregious treatments that Jeremy and others were subjected to. It also hampered a battle for recognition, rights and respect. The American activist Barbara Gittings, who fought for the deletion of homosexuality from the DSM, wrote about the impact of a diagnostic label being foisted upon a community:

> It's difficult to explain to anyone who didn't live through
> that time, how much homosexuality was under the
> thumb of psychiatry. The sickness label was an albatross

around the neck of our early gay rights groups. It
infected all our work on other issues. Anything we said
on our behalf could be dismissed as 'That's just your
sickness talking.'

As Jeremy was being assaulted with electric shocks in Yorkshire,
elsewhere campaigns to stop the practice were gathering momen-
tum. Although the medical establishment can create and hand
down a diagnosis, sometimes those labelled with it can persuasively
and powerfully shake it off.

The international movement that managed to get homosexuality
struck from the books as a mental health disorder was bolstered
by shifting legal frameworks and human rights legislation. There
was also a growing psychiatric survivor movement, and persuasive
mental health experts who themselves began to agitate for change
in a changing world. In the words of the US psychoanalyst Judd
Marmor in 1973, 'it is our task as psychiatrists to be healers of the
distressed, not watchdogs of our social mores'.

In the UK, the Counter-Psychiatry Group – part of the
Gay Liberation Front – was founded in London in 1971 by the
psychiatric social worker Elizabeth Wilson and her then partner,
the sociologist Mary McIntosh. They protested outside clinics on
Harley Street, at the Maudsley and at the Tavistock Clinic.

Meanwhile, propelled by the Stonewall riots of 1969 and the
civil rights movement that had flourished around them, gay and
lesbian activists protested at meetings of the APA. In Washington
in 1971, a 'Lifestyles of Non-Patient Homosexuals' panel invited
activists Frank Kameny and Barbara Gittings to speak. They
each outlined the stigma perpetrated by the diagnostic label of
homosexuality and later disrupted a lecture on aversion therapy,
forcing an exhibitor to stop selling picture slides used in aversion
experiments. The following year, having been invited to a panel

called 'Psychiatry: Friend or Foe to Homosexuals? A Dialogue', the activists sought to bring along a gay psychiatrist to strengthen their case – but who could come forward when their professional and personal reputation would be at stake? Their hope, Gittings remembers, was realised in the form of a man in a rubber Richard Nixon Halloween mask and oversized tuxedo:

> At last, [the psychiatrist] John Fryer said yes, provided he could wear a wig and mask and use a voice-distorting microphone. Dr. H. Anonymous was born. We smuggled him in his disguise through back corridors into the packed lecture hall. He really rocked the audience, speaking as a closeted gay person to his own colleagues, telling why he couldn't be open in his own profession.

Fryer spoke about how, in those days, gay psychiatrists had to 'know our place', and about the high price they would pay if their sexual orientation was revealed: 'We must make certain that no one in a position of power is aware of our sexual orientation or gender identity [...] lest our secret be known and our dooms sealed.'

The activists had another surprise at the dinner-dance that marked the end of the conference, when Frank Kameny brought along his date Philip Johnson, a gay activist from Dallas. 'When the band struck up a waltz, Frank and Phil sailed out onto the dance floor,' Gittings remembers. 'The other heterosexual dance couples all pretended they didn't see what they saw!'

The pivotal protests of activists, alongside growing scepticism towards traditional psychiatric approaches, the arrival of new and younger leaders at the APA, and evolving research that robustly contested a link between homosexuality and psychological maladjustment, all conspired to bring about the downfall of the diagnosis of homosexuality in the DSM and the characterisation of same-sex attraction as a mental illness.

Homosexuality was finally removed from the next reprinting of DSM-II in 1973. It was a decision that came a year after Jeremy Gavins's first meeting with the psychiatrist Hugo Milne.

It was a definitive step forwards for gay rights, for human rights; Jack Drescher pointed out that religious, government, military and educational institutes were now deprived of a medical or scientific rationalisation for discrimination.

The APA quickly denied that the protests had driven them to delete homosexuality from the DSM: its then president claimed that 'while the agitation of the gay movement quickened our sympathetic awareness of the gay concerns, the action taken was not a response to gay demands as such. It was a scientifically based decision'.*

Proceedings in the US made a difference further afield, although official change was slow to follow. Homosexuality was finally removed from the ICD in 1990. Although aversion therapy had faded from clinical practice in the UK by then, discrimination had not, even among mental health professionals. A study in the mid-1990s found a number of London psychotherapy training schools still deliberately excluding gay and lesbian trainees, in 'a web of intrigue that hovers over consulting rooms in those elegant North London suburbs [of] Islington, Hampstead and Highgate'.

As late as 2004, some British mental health professionals still defended the methods that had characterised their practice. In

---

* Although homosexuality had been removed from the DSM-II (briefly remaining as 'sexual orientation disturbance'), the term 'ego-dystonic homosexuality' lingered in DSM-III, referring to 'conflict and unhappiness about one's homosexuality and/or a desire to be heterosexual'. This was removed entirely from a revised edition of DSM-III in 1987.

an anonymous survey, one psychologist who had practised in the 1960s admitted: 'I thought they [homosexuals] were people who were disordered and needed treatment and psychiatric help. And I still do.'

The psychiatric 'disorder' of homosexuality in women was seen as distinct, in many ways, from that in men. When the BMA Committee met in 1954, they decided that in women the 'condition' could arise as a deviation in normal development 'possibly due to glandular constitution or to emotional causes'; that it tended to occur in women's prisons and remand homes, 'particularly if there is a ringleader who is a psychopathic personality or mentally subnormal'; and that it was 'one of the recognized causes of frigidity in married women'. The 'proper approach' to treating female homosexuality included 'avoidance of obvious errors in the bringing up of children'.

Research into archives from the 1960s and 1970s shows that some psychiatrists, psychotherapists and social workers encouraged women – whose homosexuality was not criminalised – to see their sexual orientation as normal and to seek out same-sex relationships. But not everyone was so lucky. Helen Spandler, Professor of Mental Health Studies at the University of Central Lancashire, who has researched the experiences of people who identify as LGBTQ+ who are psychiatric survivors, told me that at the Maudsley, a high-profile psychiatric institution, women were still being hospitalised with 'sexual deviancy' as a primary diagnosis in the 1970s.

Two decades later, Sarah Carr discovered that the medical drive to 'fix homosexuality' had not abated. Carr tells me that in 1990 she was subjected to involuntary 'reparative psychotherapy' to change her sexual orientation. She had experienced mental distress in her first year of university: 'I'd been unwell, and I thought I shouldn't be cutting myself and I shouldn't have tried to kill myself. So maybe I should get some kind of help. And I did. I went to this bloke who was a psychologist, presenting [with those symptoms].'

She expected that her mental distress would be the focus of her psychological treatment – centred around her recent relationship breakdown, her parents' reaction to her coming out ('when I was 19, they told me I wasn't to come home again'), and the stress she faced daily as a member of a minority group subject to stigma, discrimination and prejudice.

But almost two decades after Jeremy's first treatment, the diagnosis of homosexuality remained in the WHO's diagnostic manual; Sarah was suicidal and self-harming, and her therapist was certain that her sexual orientation – labelled as a psychiatric disorder – was the cause of it all. As far as he was concerned, 'it wasn't external circumstances, it was *me*, not the effects of what was going on in my life. It was actually my orientation that needed changing.'

By then, aversion therapy for same-sex attraction, at least in the way Jeremy described it, had largely become a thing of the past. But 'gay conversion therapy' or 'reparative therapy' continued to be practised internationally. In the main, electric shocks and apomorphine were supplanted by prayer, talk therapy, hypnosis and exorcism.

Sarah, still a teenager, was hypnotised by her psychologist:

> He wanted to try to coax me into a state of at
> least bisexuality, and as part of that he showed me
> pornographic pictures [of women] intended for
> heterosexual men, and asked me if I found them
> attractive or appealing or if they turned me on. I was,
> like, 'No, they don't', and he said, 'Let's try and reinforce
> that [negative] feeling through hypnotherapy.'

When that didn't turn her straight or bisexual, the psychologist decided Sarah had a personality disorder, and something traumatic, likely childhood abuse, had marked her past. 'There was something that was very fashionable at the time – repressed memory syndrome. He hypnotised me to see if he could bring any of the repressed memories forward, and it was such an unethical and such an inappropriate treatment, it was after that I absconded. He never saw me again.'

It left her distrustful of therapists for a long time: 'I would get really unwell and I would harm myself. I saw it as dealing with mental distress in a safer way.' Eventually, she found a psychotherapist she could trust, and her well-being improved, as did her relationship with her parents. 'They've become much more accepting [of the fact] that imposing those rules on me is destructive,' she says.

Sarah became an academic in the realm of mental health policy (one strand of her research examines the mental health of lesbian, gay and bisexual people), and her personal experience echoed the ones she would later come across repeatedly in the archival records of women subjected to similar treatment: the mental distress of women who happened to be attracted to the same sex was inevitably attributed to their deviant sexual orientation. These archival discoveries offered important moments of recognition. 'There's an association with being gay and being socially isolated, but I felt kind of historically isolated. I hesitate to use the word "therapeutic", but it was quite therapeutic going on that journey to meet them.'

Like Jeremy, she believes the religious establishment has much to answer for.

Sarah comes from a deeply Catholic family. Her parents were teachers at a Catholic school. 'Around the time when I was growing up, there were various papal letters that came out, I can't remember the exact phrases: sort of "homosexuality [i]s sinful", words like "vengeance".' The moral framework and ethos of the religious establishment could be neatly transposed to the medical one: both patriarchal and hierarchical, both, in her view, with dehumanising ambitions for social and moral control. 'I think it's interesting that the [DSM] is still known as the psychiatric Bible,' she says. 'In a similar way to the biblical text, they were codifying most behaviours as diagnoses, not as sins. It is a set of rules and diagnoses, to name things that are wrong with people, to have power over them and to label them, to curb socially undesirable behaviour.'

In the years after Sarah's involuntary 'reparative therapy', the psychiatric establishment relinquished its designation of homosexuality as a medical disorder, but now some religious and faith organisations have stepped back into the breach. They have leveraged and weaponised medical terminology in their efforts to 'cure homosexuality'. Sixty-nine countries still criminalise people who identify as LGBTQ+ – there and elsewhere, the shadows of those who practised aversion therapy loom, still.

Conversion therapy has been condemned by the WHO, the APA, the BMA, the Royal College of Physicians and RCPsych, the World Psychiatric Association, the AMA and many others. Some countries have imposed outright bans on these therapies, including Malta, Taiwan, Ecuador and Brazil. Moves to ban such therapies in the UK have stalled. Despite an announcement in the Queen's Speech in 2021 that the government would legislate against conversion therapy, the Government Equalities Office has stated that a consultation must be carried out first to 'ensure that the ban can address the practice while protecting the medical profession; defending freedom of speech; and upholding religious freedom'.

So for the time being at least and in many parts of the world, conversion therapy remains prevalent and sanctioned. In the US, up to a fifth of people still believe conversion therapy for young people should be legal. Some states and jurisdictions have outlawed SOCE (sexual orientation conversion efforts) by licensed practitioners. High-profile Southern Baptist leaders have denounced 'reparative therapies'. But it is still conducted by unlicensed Baptist practitioners, clergy, other spiritual advisors, and families. Nearly 700,000 'LGBT adults (ages 18–59)' have received SOCE interventions, around half of them while they were still adolescents. The Williams Institute at the UCLA School of Law predicts that, as of June 2019, '16,000 LGBT youth (ages 13–17) will receive conversion therapy from a licensed health care professional before they reach the age of 18 in the 32 states that currently do not ban the practice', and 'an estimated 57,000 LGBT youth across all states will receive conversion therapy from religious or spiritual advisors'. Extensive research shows that these methods cause lasting mental health problems including depression and suicidality, as well as internalised homophobia.

More than half of the organisations offering conversion therapy in the UK are faith groups, many invoking HIV/AIDS in their diatribes about God's wrath. In the UK, 2% of respondents to a 2017 survey of more than 100,000 people who identify as LGBTQ+ had undergone conversion therapy and 5% had been offered it.* Although the Church of England has called for a ban on conversion therapy, labelling it 'unethical [and] potentially harmful', and the Association of Christian Counsellors has also spoken out against the practice, other religious organisations

---

* The survey was 'open to anyone who identified as having a minority sexual orientation, gender identity or had variations in sex characteristics'. See *LGBT Action Plan: Improving the Lives of Lesbian, Gay, Bisexual and Transgender People* (London: Government Equalities Office, 2018).

continue to champion it. For example, the Christian organisation Core Issues Trust campaigned to be allowed to place posters reading 'Not Gay! Ex-Gay, Post-Gay and Proud. Get over it!' on London buses. After their campaign failed, their director Mike Davidson – who identifies as 'ex-gay' – said: 'We will not be intimidated or silenced. We shall continue to exercise our right freely to say that homosexual practices are unsafe for individuals, for society, and offensive to our creator God, the Lord Jesus Christ.'

The British evangelical group Christian Concern, one of the largest in the UK, believes that the campaign to ban conversion therapy has 'anti-Christian' implications and represents 'an attack on the mind of Christ'. Founder Andrea Minichiello Williams is a member of the General Synod of the Church of England and the organisation is supported by acting MPs and House of Lords peers. Hundreds of young people attend its training camps.

An undercover reporter working for the *Liverpool Echo* also recently discovered that conversion therapy was still being provided at the Anfield branch of the Mountain of Fire and Miracles Ministry. The cure would come, he was told, through a three-day programme of starvation and prayer. The ministry's global network has 90 branches across the UK. A representative later said that the organisation did not sanction practices at the church in Anfield. Its founder and General Overseer Daniel Kolawole Olukoya says that 'the Bible refers to homosexuals and lesbians as dogs' and that prayer can save those 'in the bondage [of] homosexuality, lesbianism, masturbation and prostitution'. These views are certainly not limited to conservative Christianity (the conservative or orthodox wings of many major world religions, including Islam and Judaism, pathologise anything that isn't heterosexual and doesn't conform to the gender binary), but the story of one conservative Christian organisation, Exodus International, demonstrates how this journey towards 'holier than thou' condemnation has frequently stumbled.

Once one of the largest and best known 'ex–gay' ministries in the world, Exodus was an influential lobbyist against gay marriage – its president Alan Chambers was even invited to the White House to meet with the then president George W. Bush. The organisation ran conferences to train Christian churches in how to battle the 'sin' of homosexuality, and encouraged parents to 'convert' their children to heterosexuality. The veneer began to crumble, however: Exodus co-founder Michael Busse left the group and began a relationship with another Exodus leader, Gary Cooper; and the organisation's chairman and self-proclaimed 'ex-gay' John Paulk was photographed at a gay bar in Washington DC in 2000, and later acknowledged that reparative therapy 'does great harm to many people'. Chambers himself said he had once lived a 'gay lifestyle' and continued to be attracted to other men. He issued a public apology in 2013 for the organisation's conversion practices. Although Exodus closed in 2013 after thirty-seven years in operation, its member ministries continue to operate worldwide.

Medical research and practices have partly sanctioned the conversion therapy movement within conservative Christianity and other religions. Of course, the creation of a diagnosis has the potential to drive scientific research, empower patients and deliver treatment, and patients themselves may seek out diagnosis too. But diagnoses are inescapably shrouded in the social and moral values of the time, and in a society where homophobia is common individuals like Jeremy and Sarah faced – and in many places around the world continue to face – the repercussions.

For years, Jeremy was plagued by physical symptoms – a maddening, infernal itch in his right forearm, so severe that he used wire wool sponges which stripped his skin, drew blood and left scabs, and unrelenting pains that coursed through his right arm and neck. X-rays and specialist opinions failed to yield an explanation. The symptoms disappeared when he walked the moors with his dog and when he built his beloved drystone walls.

Later, he experienced debilitating episodes in which he could barely breathe, his body trembled, his stomach cramped and flashbacks from those aversion sessions infiltrated his consciousness. During psychotherapy sessions with his counsellor, Shirley, he realised that when his body had not been able to physically escape those electric shocks as a teenager, his mind had tried to. A form of dissociation, then, which makes itself known even now.

In 2011, in one of his sessions with Shirley, he made a chilling breakthrough – maybe he hadn't seen his first love Stephen die after all. Gently, carefully, he and his therapist pieced together that the memory that had pervaded his waking hours and his worst nightmares for decades had been a false one. In truth, he had seen Stephen get off a bus many times before, and seen Stephen run across that road to meet him. But he thinks that he refashioned these truths into a falsehood in the psychiatric hospital where he was being told to erase Stephen from his mind. This was an act of psychological evasion, he explains. 'I didn't want to stop loving Stephen. I didn't want to lose him, and they – the doctors – wanted me to stop loving him. So, I'm fighting them and they're fighting me.' And somehow, he believes, all the messages got mixed up, and he imagined Stephen to be dead when he was alive. Sometime after that session he searched for Stephen online, only to discover that he had died much later, in 1983, in a car crash. He was twenty-nine years old.

Over time, the panic attacks have subsided, the physical pain too. Jeremy feels that he has finally been able to grieve Stephen. He has listened to his body, he says, and eventually understood what it was trying to tell him.

More than 15 km of drystone walls Jeremy has built over the years, he tells me with pride. He rummages about for 'me notebook', where he lists every wall he has worked on during the last two decades:

> What I've done, more or less, is build walls and that's
> where I'm happy cos I never think about anything
> but the stone. I don't get time for depression. The
> peregrines are flying in the air. The odd red squirrel
> comes bouncing past – I saw a grey squirrel t'other
> day – millions of slow worms, beautiful snakes they are,
> massive frogs, the odd lizard.

These last few weeks, the weather has been glorious. He and Timmy have been wandering over hills and swimming in rivers. 'I'm not bothered about sex or relationships and I don't think I can share what I have with somebody else,' he tells me. 'I do what I want and what makes me happy. I'm not lonely. I don't get lonely.'

He tells me that he quite likes his life now, that it took him a long time to get here but he did, and he is glad he didn't kill himself.

If the aversion therapy was supposed to banish the boy he adored from his mind, it certainly did not work. 'Back then, I found a picture in a magazine that looked a little bit like him, and on the picture I wrote, 'No matter what they do to me, I will always love you'.

Jeremy sits back a little. It takes him a moment to continue. 'I still have that magazine knocking about somewhere.'

In that picture, Stephen is forever young. On that page, their love is preserved in time. They are shielded from condemnation and vilification. Diagnosis cannot find them here, the electric shocks cannot hurt them here, the clutches of authority cannot reach them here.

'Even now, I love Stephen,' says Jeremy. 'It's ridiculous, isn't it? I'll never stop loving him.'

3

Conduct Unbecoming

'It was a vibrant neighbourhood,' Hector Pinkney remembers.
'You had shops here what were good. Everybody saying
"Morning!".' The Soho Bazaar on our left used to be a snooker
hall, he says. And before the enormous Sikh gurdwara up ahead
became a place of prayer, it was a nightclub – the Santa Rosa, the
Rialto before that.

Hector arrived in Handsworth, Birmingham from Jamaica in
1962. His father Rudolph, a cabinet maker, had landed in the UK
in 1954, followed by his wife Mavis and the rest of the family. Their
home at 68 Leonard Road was always full, Hector says. 'Eight in
our place, sometimes nine came in from next door', and whoever
else dropped in. 'My mum, she would welcome everybody.'

He pulls his green jacket a little tighter around his small frame
and rearranges his grey scarf. As the drizzle falls, he recalls the
dumplings his mother cooked for the neighbours and, later, the
blues nights that called to him each weekend.

The reggae band Steel Pulse played one of their first gigs in the
back room of the local library across the road, long before they
made the cover of the *NME*, toured with Bob Marley and won
a Grammy. Their 1978 debut album *Handsworth Revolution* was
a commentary on injustice and police racism, and a prophesy of
things to come. 'The thing was [that] then, Handsworth was a real
multicultural area,' photographer Derek Bishton tells me, as the

three of us continue our walk along Soho Road. Bishton moved here in 1975. 'There was a big white population, a big African-Caribbean population, there was a big Asian population. There was a shared sense that this was the new Britain. Handsworth was an area where all sorts of different people were rubbing along.'

We stop at the Davis Caribbean Bakery, established in 1954, the year Hector's father arrived, and take in the smell of gizzada pastries and plantain tarts, jerk wings and salt fish fritters. Along the same stretch, we pass by African Cottage, Jerk & Grill and the Little Jamaica Shop. There's a string of Asian-owned stores: Chandi Chowk, Desi Sweets, Kerala Massage and Chaii Wala, as busy as ever. And now there is also the Slovac Shop, one of a handful representing the newer waves of migrants to Handsworth. We reach the place where it all began – the site of the former Acapulco Cafe. These days, it's the Pakeeza Supermarket, but one autumn afternoon, thirty-five years ago, this modest building appeared in news bulletins across the globe.

'It was good times here until the riots came, then it all changed,' says Hector. 'The kids in Britain rebelled because they wanted change, they wanted to see change.'

The unrest that spiralled from an incident at the Acapulco Cafe had complex causes and consequences, but one lasting and bitter legacy came out of a diagnosis imposed on some of the protestors, one that was steeped in assumptions about who they were and what they were capable of. The diagnosed were predominantly African-Caribbean men who would be imprisoned, institutionalised and injected just a short distance from where we stand this morning. The diagnosis was 'cannabis psychosis', and thanks to it, as Derek puts it, 'a whole generation primarily of young men were criminalised for absolutely nothing at all'.

The diagnosis of cannabis psychosis extended to communities far beyond Handsworth, and its solid footprint remains stamped into the ones we make in this country today. Our contemporary diagnoses continue to map race onto madness and perceived hostility. One such label, as we will see in a later chapter, is increasingly being applied to children whose futures are determined by it, leaving them, at once, at risk of medicalisation and criminalisation. We have an opportunity not to repeat the same mistakes in our schools and hospitals today that were made on the streets of Handsworth more than thirty-five years ago. By revisiting and learning from the past, we could hope to change our future.

At 4.45 p.m. on 9 September 1985, a police officer discovered a car parked without a tax disc by the junction of Villa Road and Lozells Road. A chief constable's report later stated that the driver, when confronted, gave a false address, became aggressive, was arrested, and then broke away and ran into the nearby Acapulco Cafe. 'A large number of Black youths gathered,' the report goes on to say. Converging police officers came under attack. One was kicked from his bike. Others faced 'stones, bottles and staves as they attempted to arrest those responsible'. Eleven police officers were injured and seven vehicles were damaged.

Some said the violence was hardly one-sided. A witness later told an independent investigation that a black woman who tried to intervene was punched by an officer and knocked to the ground. This woman never came forward, and the account remains uncorroborated.

What everybody agrees on, though, is that tensions escalated rapidly. By 7.35 p.m., the Bingo Hall at Villa Cross was in flames. Within twenty-five minutes, more than 200 people had gathered near Villa Cross and missiles were being thrown at firefighters and police officers. At Lozells Road, a few hundred yards away, fire bombs were launched into a shopping centre. By 8.30 p.m., several burning cars lay overturned, and the firefighters had been forced to retreat under a hail of bricks and stones. Looters appeared with bolt cutters and crowbars. By 9 p.m., 500 people were milling around on Villa Road, facing around the same number of police. Masonry fell as buildings continued to burn. By 4 a.m., the fire brigade finally gained access and most of the crowd dissipated. It seemed that the worst was over.

But in fact the unrest raged on for a further two days. The news emerged that two brothers who ran the post office had died during the evening of 9 September. At 8.58 p.m., police had received a phone call from the Moledina bothers – Kassamali, aged thirty-eight, and Amirali, aged forty-four – with the message 'Please help, they are smashing their way in, they want to kill us'. Later, it was confirmed that the brothers had succumbed to smoke inhalation, but in the moment rumours swirled and accusations mounted. A false account appeared in the *Sun* newspaper, which claimed that 'Two Asian brothers screamed in agony as West Indian rioters beat them – and left them to burn alive in the petrol-bombed sub-post office.'

On 10 September, the Conservative Home Secretary Douglas Hurd visited Handsworth and came under attack when a crowd of several hundred people – described by an independent report as '95% Black, including some Rastafarians with some Whites and Asians' – started hurling bricks in his direction. He was bundled away from the scene. Skirmishes continued, more petrol bombs and bricks were thrown, shops broken into and set on fire. The post office in Rookery Road was raided, and the postmaster's wife held by the neck and threatened.

By 11 September, the Handsworth riots had made international headlines, with *The New York Times* reporting that 'the neighborhood looked as if it had been bombed from the air, with roofs and walls collapsed [...] the horror grew as two badly charred bodies were found in a post office'. The West Midlands police chief constable Geoffrey Dear 'thought it was possible that recent television news pictures of riots by blacks in South Africa had encouraged the mob here'.

That evening, police and community leaders came together to draw up plans aimed at restoring the peace. Over the next few hours, calm was returned to the streets. After three days of violence, two men had died; 35 civilians and 79 police officers had been injured, alongside eight firefighters and paramedics; and 145 people had been arrested.

But the origins of the troubles in Handsworth went far deeper than those headlines could ever suggest.

To understand the riots, Derek Bishton tells me, you have to understand what Handsworth was like back then. By 1985, it had become the most socially deprived area in Britain, with the highest unemployment rate and notoriously overcrowded housing. *The New York Times* described it as 'a neighborhood of dilapidated homes and shops with heavy security grills [...] of 16,000 homes, some 15,000 have neither a bath nor a toilet'.

Deindustrialisation and deep recession had taken their toll on the broader West Midlands region with a loss of 25% of manufacturing jobs between 1978 and 1981, more than 4,000 of those in Handsworth. At the time of the riots, unemployment was at 38% – nearly double the average of the city of Birmingham and three times the national rate. In the area immediately surrounding the riots, there were 3,500 unemployed young people, at a time when a third of employers openly admitted to discriminating against black applicants. 'Black youth had no future,' says Hector Pinkney. 'They got no future now.'

Relations between police and the community were strained. 'We could not stand on the street and have a conversation,' remembers Hector. '"You're not allowed here, son," they'd say. "Get back to your

end.'"The 'sus law' – as the Vagrancy Act 1824 was then nicknamed
– had given police discretionary power to arrest anyone suspected
of loitering with intent to commit an arrestable offence. The act
was a Victorian relic targeting 'idle and disorderly persons'; under
its auspices, a black person was 15 times more likely to be arrested
than someone who was white. An underclass of black people in the
most deprived areas of the inner city were being unjustly marked
out, the Institute of Race Relations reported in 1979, and forced
to battle against a charge that was virtually impossible to rebut.
'Sus' was repealed in 1981, but then effectively reinstated as a 'stop
and search' power by the time of the 1985 Handsworth riots, by
the Police and Criminal Evidence Act 1984; a simple 'reasonable
suspicion' was the only requirement.

Derek (who is white) witnessed these sorts of injustices as he
photographed the riots:

> I was put in the cells in Thornhill Road. They knew I
> was a journalist and photographer and so I was treated
> quite well, I wasn't physically attacked. But while I was
> waiting, in the cell next to me somebody got battered. I
> mean absolutely battered. The poor guy was just numbed
> senseless. For years, many were criminalised for nothing
> more than walking on the streets.

As an independent inquiry led by barrister and former Labour MP
Julius Silverman concluded in 1986, the riots spoke for 'a frustrated
and angry group who have suffered over a long period of time
and are generally alienated from society'. Racial discrimination
represented, as Silverman put it, 'part of the alienation felt by
ethnic communities and in my view it is an essential element in
the cause of the riots'.

But at the time, and in the weeks following, the press reported the riots from a very different angle. 'Wild Ganja Linked to the Riots: Dangerous Habit Spreading Among Blacks' ran the headline in the *Birmingham Evening Mail* in early October: 'Ganja, a form of cannabis, had a direct bearing on events in Birmingham's riot-scarred multi-racial suburb, West Birmingham Health Authority experts believe.' A report to the health authority drew explicit links between 'ganja intoxication', psychosis and violence.

This was reportedly an epidemic of sorts, with the regional drug addiction unit at All Saints' Hospital under pressure to cope with 'more and more cases of ganja junkies'. Local health centres were 'bursting at the seams' trying to help patients at risk of developing cannabis psychosis, and a rehabilitation centre was urgently needed, along with research to understand Handsworth's drug issues. The violence, said Birmingham's Lord Mayor, was 'absolute thuggery gone mad on drugs'. Media reports had reduced the protestors to senseless, drug-fuelled aggressors, a depiction enabled and empowered by the pre-existing and then widely accepted diagnostic label of cannabis psychosis, which had been frequently used within policing and medical circles to explain the behaviour of those who were disenfranchised and marginalised. The linking of race, madness and drugs has deep cultural roots. Handsworth provided a fertile soil in which those roots could take hold.

Cannabis products (ganja, hashish, marijuana, bhang, charas) have long been blamed for inciting violence, but much of the English-language literature on this presumptive connection came from British medical men and politicians in India in the nineteenth century. 'When an Indian wants to commit some horrible crime, such as murder or wife mutilation,' wrote the MP William Caine in 1890, 'he prepares himself for it with two annas' worth of bhang from a government majoon shop.' In 1893, the Indian Hemp Drugs Commission assessed more than 2,300 patients at 24 asylums and concluded that moderate use usually had 'no injurious effect on the mind', although for those with a pre-existing mental disorder, or a vulnerability to one, 'it may be accepted as reasonably proved, in the absence of evidence of other cause, that hemp drugs do cause insanity'.

The insanity in men (women were generally believed to be spared of it) could be short- or long-lived and could persist even after drug use had ceased. The brutality of which they were capable was striking, as reported by Major G. F. W. Ewens, superintendent at the Punjab Lunatic Asylum in 1904. Ewens was especially concerned about the use of charas, which he described as the most concentrated form of hemp plants, smoked or swallowed whole: 'I am not aware of any men addicted to excess of charas who have remained sane.'

Here are two case studies from Ewens' records:

> *Sunder Singh, admitted 24th June 1900, [aged] 20.* – [...]
> [D]irty, noisy, destructive to clothing, went naked. [...]
> Became demented and a mud eater. Still in the asylum.
> The father states that his insanity followed his habits of
> indulgence in charas.

> *Jan Mahamad, admitted 27th September 1900, [aged] 45.* –
> A beggar admitted as a criminal lunatic having savagely
> assaulted without provocation three British soldiers at
> Peshawar. He has a history of excess in charas, etc. [...]
> Delusions as to having his land stolen from him. [...]
> Still at the asylum, improved, quiet but weak-minded.

Reports linking cannabis and insanity emerged throughout the twentieth century, usually focused on its acute effects – short-lived marijuana-induced madness in stoned soldiers in Vietnam or in unruly prisoners. Descriptions of *chronic* psychosis, however, were invariably limited to patients in India and North Africa, and often written up by European and North American doctors stationed there. It was framed as a sort of local madness, one that Europeans and Americans were suspiciously immune to. In a 1966 report on cannabis psychosis in Moroccan patients, their 'severe disorientation as to time' was attributed to a culturally specific 'traditional cultural disregard for time in Morocco'. Case studies of chronic psychosis in patients in the UK began to surface only in the 1970s and 1980s, and even then the studies were mainly concerned with African-Caribbean people.

Yet eighty years after Ewens described the condition in his patients at Punjab Lunatic Asylum there was still no medical consensus in Britain on what cannabis psychosis actually *was*. It was not a formal diagnosis decided upon by medical committees with an accepted list of criteria and recorded in textbooks. Instead, when a psychiatrist identified a patient as psychotic – that is, expressing false perceptions (hallucinations) and false beliefs (delusions and paranoia) – the diagnosis was cannabis psychosis if cannabis use could be directly linked to the patient's symptoms. There was not even any agreement on how best to confirm such a direct link. What form of cannabis might precipitate it, and how much? What if a patient had taken cannabis a week or a month before – could the drug still be responsible? How could cannabis psychosis be differentiated from acute cannabis intoxication or schizophrenia (another condition of psychosis)? If a psychotic patient stopped taking cannabis and remained psychotic, was the diagnosis still cannabis psychosis? In a 1988 survey of more than a hundred psychiatrists, poor concentration was accepted as a symptom by only around 60%. A suggested list of five psychiatric features for the condition (poor concentration, delusions of persecution, auditory hallucinations, clouding of consciousness and agitation) was not accepted by around half of those questioned. Not all psychiatrists even supported the idea that there was a relationship between cannabis and psychosis in the first place.

In fact, long-standing research on whether cannabis causes psychosis has yielded conflicting results. Some contemporary studies suggest people diagnosed with psychosis are more likely to report current or prior use of the drug, but association and cause are not the same thing. As Carl Hart of Columbia University and Charles Ksir of the University of Wyoming have said:

> In our many decades of college teaching, one of the most important things we have tried to impart to our students is the distinction between correlation (two things are statistically associated) and causation (one thing causes another). For example, the wearing of light clothing is more likely during the same months as higher sales of ice-cream, but we do not believe that either causes the other.

Along the same lines, a Missouri study examining the records of 158 psychiatric admissions found that 38 of these were preceded by marijuana use, 94 by dancing, and 123 by watching a late-night film. Other variables that produced higher 'hit rates' than marijuana for psychotic episodes included masturbation and sex education. If you decide cannabis is responsible for inciting madness, shouldn't you blame dancing and films and masturbation and sex education too?

The truth is that any link between cannabis and psychosis is likely to be highly nuanced. Seemingly significant associations uncovered to date could simply represent the possibility of a shared genetic risk for psychosis and propensity towards cannabis use. In other words, some people might carry a genetic blueprint that makes them vulnerable to *both* factors (A: cannabis use, B: psychosis), rather than A *causing* B.

What has been consistent about the diagnosis of cannabis psychosis, however, is its racialised nature. The association between drugs, madness, violence and specifically race was strongly promoted in the US throughout the 1930s by Harry J. Anslinger, commissioner of the Federal Bureau of Narcotics. He labelled it 'the most violence-causing drug in the history of mankind', and invoked race in his claim that 'most marijuana smokers are Negroes, Hispanics, jazz musicians, and entertainers. Their satanic music is driven by marijuana, and marijuana smoking by white women makes them want to seek sexual relations with Negroes, entertainers, and others.'

The tabloid press in the UK was drawn towards these racialised depictions, which they illustrated with pictures of smoke-filled drug dens, patronised by users invariably depicted as Chinese or Arab, next to semi-naked white British women who had seemingly fallen prey to the vices of these foreign interlopers with their corrupting opium and marijuana. This supposed threat to the purity of the nation's women was reflected in the ominous words of John Ralph in the *Sunday Graphic* in 1951:

> We are dealing with the most evil men who have ever
> taken to the vice business. The victims are teenage
> British girls, and to a lesser extent, teenage youths [...]
> the racketeers are 90 per cent coloured men from the
> West Indies and west coast of Africa [...] there is greatest
> danger of the reefer craze becoming the greatest social
> menace this country has known.

In this state of racialised moral panic, cannabis legislation could be used to criminalise and marginalise minorities, who were already seen as a menace to existing moral standards and social cohesion.

At the time of the Handsworth riots, this line was still being drawn between cannabis and psychosis, in black men in particular. Yet there was no good evidence to suggest African-Caribbean men were smoking more cannabis – in fact, some studies at the time suggested white men were more likely to do so.* Some of the black men who formally received a diagnosis of cannabis psychosis in Handsworth argued they had never even used cannabis, and one psychiatrist's review of their notes found that the condition was sometimes diagnosed even when their urine had not been tested for the drug. When cannabis *was* present, there was little evidence it had caused psychosis, let alone any lingering mental health effects at all.

The ganja of the 1980s may have been a different substance to the cannabis we see on the streets today; comparing the potency of today's drugs and those of the 1980s is impossible – laboratory testing of ganja potency was infrequent then, and drew on different scientific methods. Contemporary studies that point to associations between cannabis and psychosis refer to high-potency or heavy daily cannabis use; research on current drugs cannot be extrapolated to past ones. Despite this, cannabis psychosis was a diagnosis easily imposed on black men in Handsworth. In a 1988 UK survey, 59 of 82 psychiatrists believed cannabis psychosis was more common in 'people of Afro-Caribbean origin (West Indians)'. The following year, twelve psychiatrists ('ten of UK origin, one

---

* These results were replicated in the 2016 Home Office *Crime Survey for England and Wales*, according to which Black or Black British young men were twice less likely than white young men to have used cannabis in the last year. Those from mixed heritage backgrounds were 1.5 times more likely to have smoked cannabis in the same time period (Home Office, 'Drug Misuse: Findings from the 2015/16 *Crime Survey for England and Wales*', 28 Jul 2016).

of Caribbean and one of Asian origin') agreed that virtually all patients with a diagnosis of cannabis psychosis were men and two thirds or more were African-Caribbean. They also claimed, contrary to the evidence, that African-Caribbeans tended to use cannabis more often and in larger amounts than other groups. The association was so strong that one psychiatrist questioned in the survey commented that if a black youth of around 20 with an 'Afro-Caribbean haircut came in "out of his mind" one naturally tended to diagnose "cannabis psychosis"'. This approach was seen elsewhere too: a 1982 study in South Africa examined the condition only in 'every third consecutive Cape Coloured man' admitted to the Valkenberg psychiatric hospital, even though the racially segregated hospital also had white patients.

Suman Fernando, a psychiatrist in North London at that time and a long-standing critic of the diagnosis, tells me that in the 1980s 'if you were black, they would in the first instance look for cannabis. It was so inbred in the psychiatric system'. He analysed a series of case notes in his own hospital back then, and discovered that it was primarily black patients who were subjected to cannabis testing. 'We discussed it at the ward round, and I said, "I've looked at the statistics – we ought to do testing on everyone if we do it." That was taken to heart, but six to eight months later, nothing had changed.'

The diagnosis was seldom made in Birmingham in the early to mid-1970s. By the early 1980s, however, over a quarter of second-generation African-Caribbean psychiatric patients aged 16–29 in central Birmingham were labelled with cannabis psychosis. In white men of the same age, the figure was 1%. The diagnoses more commonly made in white and Asian patients with psychosis, regardless of whether or not they had used cannabis in the recent or remote past, were bipolar disorder and schizophrenia.

Because the diagnosis of cannabis psychosis was already heavily racialised, it was easy to apply to the Handsworth protestors, especially when the press was already presenting the riots through a racist lens. The *Daily Express* reported on 'Zulu-style war cries'. *The Sun* described the riots as 'tribal'. A photograph of a young black man carrying a lit petrol bomb was used in the *Daily Express*, *Daily Mirror*, *Observer* and *Daily Mail*. In *The Sun*, the same photo was captioned in an incendiary manner: 'A black thug stalks a Birmingham street with hate in his eyes and a petrol bomb in his hand. The prowling West Indian was one of the hoodlums who brought new race terror to the city's riot-torn Handsworth district yesterday.'

The same newspaper published these words under the headline 'Song of joy by rioters':

> Whooping West Indians sang 'Oh, What A Beautiful
> Morning' as they surveyed the riot wreckage yesterday.
> They laughed and drank while one section of the
> community mourned the victims of the violence. And
> they jeered and booed Police and firemen dealing with
> the burnt out cars littering a stretch of road nick-named
> Mayhem Mile.

TV coverage of the riots carried footage of men (the voiceover describing them as 'West Indian youths') smoking marijuana.

These reports failed to convey, often wilfully so, the broad make-up of the crowds. The Silverman Inquiry report concluded that

> not all the rioters were black and certainly not all the
> looters were black. The proportion varied at different
> places and at different times. Although the majority
> was black on the Lozells Road, there were a significant

number of white rioters – probably 20–25%. There
was also a small percentage of Asians. Indeed this was a
multi-racial riot.

The New York Times reported that 'the presence of so many whites
in court made it appear that the carnage in Handsworth might
be yet another manifestation of the kind of violence that Britain
has frequently suffered at the hands of unruly soccer fans'. The
journalist watched each one step up to the dock. Colin Leacy,
first of all, a white civil servant from Aston accused of setting fire
to a car, theft and threatening behaviour. And then John Sheehy,
'a white accused of throwing rocks at the police'.

The multi-racial nature of the riots wasn't only a feature of
Handsworth. Of those arrested for riot-related offences across
London in 1981, the largest single group (accounting for one
third) was white. Although the Toxteth riots of 1981 were related
to the arrest of a young black motorcyclist, the arrest data points
to a heterogeneous population: as many as 60% were white. The
Moss Side rioters in Manchester that same year included 'a large
minority of Whites'. The investigative journalist Tony Bunyan
wrote that 'the black community and the dispossessed white
working class, living side by side in the squalid ghetto areas of
Britain's major cities, joined together to fight the police – the
common denominator and symbol of their oppression.'

The diagnosis of cannabis psychosis itself has indisputable
shortcomings, and these led to its being deployed almost effortlessly
in discriminatory ways. The medical establishment's imprimatur
gave 'cannabis psychosis' legitimacy, even as some in the profession
sought to deny its existence. In the press, the Handsworth riots
were reduced to the spectre of mentally unstable drug-fuelled
black men stirring up trouble. According to this view, angry
young black men who had the audacity to protest could have

no justifiable reason to do so. Their rage was symptomatic of a medical disturbance, it was pathological, it was psychiatric, it was criminal. It was not legitimate.

Less than a mile away from the din of Birmingham's Soho Road, it's a crisp afternoon, and peaceful. A faint gurgle from the canal nearby, the breeze has dropped, the drizzle has disappeared. A tow path curves around the southern boundary of a grey-walled Victorian Gothic prison. Next to it stands an old asylum building with a gloomy brick facade, acres of green space rolling away around it. Both prison and asylum were designed by the same architect. The asylum, later renamed All Saints' Hospital, first opened in 1850. A patient recalled an early Christmas Eve party there in 1853: 'Nearly two hundred of God's erring and deeply afflicted children, called lunatics, assembled clean, neat, quiet with at least a passing smile on their careworn and in some cases half-conscious countenances; a decided cheerfulness, nay merriment on some, and on others an expression of pleasing astonishment.'

Both Derek and Hector heard less than glowing accounts of the place in the 1980s. 'It was something out of Dickens,' says Derek:

> It was the typical lunatic asylum set in beautiful grounds
> and built on what was then the outside of the city.
> Mental health care was terrible them, it was quite
> draconian and there was much less sympathy for mental
> illness in the community. People were sectioned and had
> absolutely no rights.

There was a connecting channel between it and the prison, he remembers. 'You could take people out without going out of the establishment – straight from the prison to the hospital.' A bell used to go off whenever someone escaped, Hector tells me, easily heard across the town. 'If you rebel,' he says, 'you guarantee you're going to get the juk [the syringe that carried a powerful tranquiliser].'

It's impossible to establish with absolute certainty how many people were diagnosed with cannabis psychosis in the days and weeks around the riots, but it is clear that the diagnosis was applied to more black men in the area than white and Asian men in the preceding years. Of 72 West Indian men (as categorised by researchers at the time) detained at All Saints' – the local psychiatric hospital for Handsworth – more than 10% received this diagnosis between 1975 and 1982. These years were marked by growing social deprivation, unrest, and an earlier riot in 1981. Of the 420 white men who were detained in the same time frame, not a single one received a diagnosis of cannabis psychosis.*

In the immediate aftermath of the riots, the number diagnosed with cannabis psychosis rose sharply. Newspapers drew on health authority reports to claim that All Saints' was under remarkable strain to manage a mounting number of patients with the diagnosis, as were local health centres who referred their patients onwards to All Saints'. Once the violence of the riots had dissipated, though, the diagnosis of cannabis psychosis in Birmingham began to vanish too. Three years after the riots, psychiatrists at All Saints' wrote to the *BMJ* to say that they had not diagnosed a single person with cannabis psychosis for more than three months. Perhaps a medical label to describe the violence of rioting black men was no longer expedient. But those who had already received the diagnosis, I discovered, continued to be injected with tranquilisers long after the diagnostic label disappeared from their communities.

*

---

* Racial and ethnic grouping differed between studies at the time. In this study, 'West Indian' included 'migrant' and 'British' groups.

While cannabis and madness had long been linked, what changed in the early 1980s was the willingness of at least some in the medical establishment to apply the diagnostic label of cannabis psychosis liberally. There was no justification for the disproportionate application of this label to black men, and yet it sanctioned the harsh medical interventions that followed. The diagnosis was characterised by bias; its treatments were too.

Most of the hundred or so psychiatrists questioned in a 1988 study agreed that cannabis psychosis, if it was indeed a diagnosis, was a self-limiting condition (i.e. one that could resolve spontaneously, without medication), yet paradoxically 70% thought that 'major tranquilisers' were the most appropriate treatment.

That the 'treatment of choice' was so extreme is not surprising. African-Caribbean men in the British mental health system, regardless of diagnosis, were much less likely to be offered psychotherapy and more likely to receive drugs and electroconvulsive therapy at the time, even if they shared the same symptoms of psychosis as white patients. These disparities in treatment were echoed in other parts of Europe and in North America. There was also a disturbing distinction in the type of drug they received. A 'depot' is a slow-release, slow-acting injection form of an antipsychotic, frequently given to patients deemed 'non-compliant'. In one East London study conducted in 1985, men born in the Caribbean were more likely to receive 'depot injections' than those born in the UK, even though almost all expressed a preference for tablets rather than injections, often repeatedly so. This was also the case, albeit to a lesser extent, for Caribbean-born women. A depot prescription meant these patients were 'tied to the system', requiring attendance at a clinic rather than being able to take tablets at home. A reluctance to accept injections over tablets was seen as an informed choice in white patients, but in black patients it was evidence of irrationality, if not insanity. The medical staff who prescribed and administered these injections were enacting, even if unconsciously, selective control of these black men and women judged to be difficult and defiant. It might have been medically prescribed chemical suppression rather than legally enforced sanction, but the end results were chillingly similar – the overpowering and punishment of people incarcerated in systems that discriminated against them in every encounter.

Another survey from Nottingham found that African-Caribbean patients were not only more likely to be prescribed depot antipsychotic injections, they also received higher peak doses, which increased the chances of the patient experiencing debilitating long-term toxicity. They were more likely to develop somnolence, weight gain, sexual dysfunction, and a Parkinson's-type syndrome of extreme slowing down – walking reduced to an unsteady shuffle, rigidity in the arms and legs, and an incapacitating involuntary tremor. Some were left with tardive dyskinesia – a highly visible and stigmatising syndrome that is caused by these antipsychotics and characterised by repetitive and rhythmic movements of facial grimacing, chewing, tongue protrusion, eye blinking, grunting, smacking of the lips and writhing of the limbs – symptoms that were frequently irreversible even if the antipsychotics were withdrawn.

In summary, black men, who were already more likely to be detained, were also more likely to be diagnosed with cannabis psychosis and more likely to be injected with potent, possibly life-changing antipsychotics.

Derek told me that men from the local community would be

> remanded for a short while, and if they were considered to be a problem, this ganja psychosis diagnosis was used to drug them and effectively release them back into the communities as zombies. Once you had been in that system you couldn't get out of it. You had to attend

for your next injection or you were arrested. If you
tried resisting arrest because you didn't like what was
happening, you were in more trouble, and so on and on
it went. It was a vicious circle.

Cannabis psychosis had sealed the fate of these men. The diagnosis
compromised their care within the mental health system and
jeopardised their future outside it. All Saints' closed in 2000 (the
prison next to it remains open).

Even if the diagnosis of cannabis psychosis has faded from the
streets of Handsworth, even if the old asylum has closed, it has left
its mark on the police patrolling the streets elsewhere.

During a year of fieldwork leading up to the 2011 riots in South
and East London, the researcher Daniel Bear of Humber College
in Toronto, spent 600 hours with street-level police officers in a
pseudonymous inner London borough:

Officers were almost to a person convinced that drug
[cannabis] use would cause serious psychological
problems. Many, even those that were not opposed to
legalizing cannabis believed that, 'Skunk rots your brain.
The chemicals, the smoke; brings on psychosis before
you can even say "Rastafarian"' (PC Henry). 'Yeah, you
get that brown brain with cannabis' (PC Rosanne, RT2).
This logic did not preclude an officer from being pro
[the] legalisation or decriminalization of cannabis, it
was simply seen as a problem associated with the drug.
As one officer put it, 'We're coming down hard on soft
minds' (PC Green).

Aside from the fact that cannabis has not been proven to cause
psychosis, not all cannabis products are made equal. Some, like 'super

skunk', have much higher levels of THC (tetrahydrocannabinol, which accounts for the drug's psychoactive effects) than home-grown skunk, hash or weed. The assumption that today's more readily available super-strength forms of cannabis must lead to psychosis has been countered by findings that a dramatic increase in marijuana use over the past fifty years has not been associated with increased rates of psychosis over the same period. I'm struck by those racialised overtones that go beyond the strength or sort of cannabis – the stereotypical depiction of a 'Rastafarian psychotic' brings to mind the same judgements made decades ago in Birmingham.

Diagnoses of cannabis psychosis implied certain beliefs about behaviour – the drug-fuelled black man in Handsworth, defined by deep-seated assumptions about who he was and what he was capable of. The chronicle of cannabis psychosis is not one that can be safely relegated to history, even if we no longer see tabloid headlines describing 'Zulu-style war cries' and 'prowling West Indian[s]'.

The psychiatrist Suman Fernando tells me that the term 'cannabis psychosis' fell out of use as a common explanation for delusions and hallucinations because it came to be seen as racist. Another diagnosis replaced it, he says. While cases of cannabis psychosis waned, 'the number of black people who were diagnosed with schizophrenia went up'. Schizophrenia is a condition marked by severe psychiatric symptoms such as auditory hallucinations, paranoid delusions and disorganised speech and behaviour. These symptoms typically develop in later adolescence or early adulthood, and usually last months rather than weeks if untreated.

Cannabis psychosis still exists in APA and WHO classification manuals,* but the debate continues regarding whether cannabis can cause ongoing psychosis, or whether an apparent diagnosis of cannabis psychosis might simply represent a first episode of schizophrenia. A recent Danish study found that around 40% of patients with an initial diagnosis of cannabis psychosis 'converted' to schizophrenia over 20 years. Half did so within 3 years, but the other half did so after many more years, suggesting that the initial label of cannabis psychosis could have been a misdiagnosis.†

Schizophrenia quickly became a diagnosis that selectively marked the same men in the UK who had been labelled as stoned psychotics before. In 1988, psychiatrists at All Saints' reported on the diagnoses of 210 patients admitted over a three-month period. None received a diagnosis of cannabis psychosis, not even those who had been detained under the Mental Health Act. Seventy per cent of 'Afro-Caribbean' patients received a diagnosis of schizo-phrenia or a related diagnosis called schizoaffective disorder (in which a mood disorder such as depression accompanies psychosis), compared to 57% of 'Asian patients' and 29% 'of British origin' ('British origin' seems to have been synonymous with 'white').

This racialised application of schizophrenia emerged in the US decades before it reached Britain. There, the diagnosis was affixed to allegedly violent, belligerent black men who rebelled

---

* It is now termed 'cannabis-induced psychotic disorder' or 'cannabis abuse with psychotic disorder'. Cannabis-induced psychosis is typically said to develop within a week of cannabis use, usually during periods of heavy substance use or a sudden increase in cannabis potency.

† Could cannabis use have triggered later schizophrenia in these patients? There is no definitive evidence to support this. Instead, social, environmental and genetic factors that increase the likelihood of using cannabis could be the same ones that increase the chance of developing schizophrenia.

and rioted, to Black Panthers and Black Power, even to those who dared to question entrenched inequalities or seek change. Doctors made the diagnosis; the FBI did so too, readily. But it hadn't always been this way. In the US, during the first half of the twentieth century, schizophrenia was a condition of mildly unhappy young white women. The dramatic alteration in the poster patient for schizophrenia – from docile young white woman to antagonistic black man – set the scene for its importation to our shores.

From the 1920s to the 1950s, schizophrenia was seen in American medical and popular opinion as primarily a disease of white people. It was characterised in academic articles and at conferences as a state of 'emotional disharmony', one of indifference but not invective. The *Ladies' Home Journal* and *Better Homes and Gardens* described its typical patient: an unhappily married middle-class white woman with 'Dr Jekyll and Mrs Hyde' mood swings. Case notes included comments such as 'this patient wasn't able to take care of her family as she should'; 'this patient is not well adjusted and can't do her housework'; 'she got confused and talked too loudly and embarrassed her husband'. Therapy recommendations included gardening, basket weaving and pottery. In 1935, *The New York Times* cautioned that the 'grandiloquence' of poets and novelists was 'one of the telltale phrases of schizophrenia, the mild form of insanity known as split personality'. If crime was involved at all, it was usually of the petty and non-violent sort. The 1952 definition of schizophrenia in the DSM only hinted coyly at 'unpredictable behavior'.

Over the following two decades, however, schizophrenia was recast as a form of mental illness displayed by activists in the civil rights movement; this changing picture is deftly outlined by psychiatrist Jonathan Metzl in his book *Protest Psychosis*. Men associated with Black Power, the Black Panthers and the Nation of Islam were particularly vulnerable. Two New York psychiatrists writing in the *Archives of General Psychiatry* in 1968 reported that black men fighting for civil rights developed 'hostile and aggressive feelings' and 'delusional anti-whiteness', a syndrome they termed as 'protest psychosis'. The madness of these men was, Walter Bromberg and Franck Simon wrote, 'guided in content by African subcultural ideologies and colored by a denial of Caucasian values and hostility'. It was 'virtually a repudiation of white civilization'. These young men often drew pictures or wrote material 'of Islamic nature', adopted 'Islamic names', drew on African ideology 'with a decided "primitive" accent' and revelled in the language 'of basic voodooism'. Their abject anger lay at the heart of this disorder and their call for justice was deemed pathological: 'Their statements appear to be bizarre in the extreme and patently dramatized, often outlandish.' The threat to the existing establishment was grave: 'The psychotic productions merge into utterances of those Moslems (in the USA) who advocate no less than dethronement of the traditional evaluation of white supremacy in religion and culture.'

The FBI labelled Malcolm X as having 'pre-psychotic paranoid schizophrenia'. Robert Williams of the NAACP (the National Association for the Advancement of Colored People) was 'schizophrenic, armed, and dangerous', they reported. A *Chicago Tribune* headline in July 1966 read 'FBI adds Negro mental patient to "10 most wanted" list', describing Leroy Ambrosia Frazier as 'an extremely dangerous and mentally unbalanced schizophrenic escapee from a mental institution, who has a lengthy criminal record and history of violent assaults'.

The perceived 'hostility' and 'aggression' of black men, whether they had participated in riots or not, neatly mapped onto the diagnostic descriptors of schizophrenia that were evolving in parallel at the APA. By 1968, after many meetings and drafts in the years since its first edition in 1952, their updated DSM-II carried a new profile of a typical paranoid schizophrenic, as intimidating and defiant: 'The patient's attitude is frequently hostile and aggressive and his behavior tends to be consistent with his delusions.' Even black men hospitalised for decades with another psychiatric diagnosis (such as a personality disorder) now found themselves labelled with schizophrenia. Conversely, the basket-weaving schizophrenic white woman sometimes was re-diagnosed as melancholic or neurotic.*

An edgy racist iconography grew up around this burgeoning diagnosis of the hostile, aggressive schizophrenic and the medications on offer to treat him. In the 1950s, advertisements for Serpasil (reserpine) showed women serenely sewing and reading. By the 1970s, advertisements for Haldol, another antipsychotic, depicted a belligerent black man, clenched fist raised in the air. The setting was an urban one, the windows behind him carried the orange reflections of burning buildings. The text read: 'Assaultive and belligerent? Cooperation often begins with Haldol.' Advertisements for the antipsychotic Thorazine led with 'Basic tools of primitive psychiatry', adding photographs of Africanised icons, as if there was any doubt as to who these primitives were. Sales materials for Stelazine (trifluoperazine) featured pictures of tribal artefacts and masks.

By the 1960s, the National Institute of Mental Health reported that 'blacks have a 65% higher rate of schizophrenia than whites'. In the 1970s, researchers found that not only were African Americans

---

* Metzl believes that the explanation for a dramatic detour in the definition of schizophrenia went far beyond the racist intentions of individual doctors. Instead, he writes in *Protest Psychosis*, it reflected the social environment in which it was produced, one infiltrated by 'growing cultural anxieties about social change'.

significantly more likely to receive a diagnosis of schizophrenia than white patients, they were less likely to receive other mental health diagnoses such as depression or bipolar disorder. Similar patterns began to emerge in the UK in the same decade: rates of schizophrenia in 'West Indians' were three to five times that seen in 'Whites', even when accounting for age and social class. British-born children of migrants from the West Indies consistently had even higher first admission rates for schizophrenia than their parents' generation.

This over-representation persists today. In England, the risk of being diagnosed with schizophrenia remains higher for all minority ethnic groups, but particularly so for Black Africans, who are nearly six times more likely to be diagnosed with schizophrenia than a white English patient. Black Caribbean people are around five times more likely to receive the diagnosis than a white British patient.* Across the UK, the incidence for schizophrenia in Black Caribbean people is among the highest in the world, far exceeding rates in Jamaica, Barbados and Trinidad. In the US, African American men are up to four times more likely to be diagnosed with schizophrenia than white patients.

In all these studies of mental health in the UK and beyond, even the very concepts of race and ethnicity are complex. Racial categories have frequently constructed 'biological reality' where

---

* All studies cited in this chapter use varying descriptors for ethnic and racial groups. I've replicated their terms used for consistency within studies. In the one I've mentioned above, 'South Asians', 'White Other' and 'Mixed Ethnicity' were also at moderately higher risk (RR 2.27, 2.24 and 2.24 respectively). The 'White Other' category in this research included people born in countries where the majority population is 'White' (e.g. Poland, Ireland, Germany). This contrasted with 'White British', which included people who were UK-born or UK-born Europeans.

there is none. Inconsistent terminology is characteristic: 'West Indian', 'Black', 'Afro-Caribbean' or 'African-descended' have been used interchangeably. I've quoted verbatim the categories and capitalisations researchers used so as to reflect their findings as they saw them, contemporaneous with events of the time, but in these categories, culture, race, skin colour and ethnicity are frequently conflated. Race, itself a social construct, frequently fails to map onto the terms people use to self-identify.

No single biological or genetic reason explains the over-representation of schizophrenia diagnoses in different ethnic or racial groups, but what these studies can tell us – their flawed racial and ethnic categorisations notwithstanding – is that some groups are collectively disadvantaged. The factors that mark out social disadvantage (homelessness, poverty and deprivation, lack of social support and unemployment) are also those that drive an increased risk of mental health issues.*

We are left with the perception of the typical schizophrenic patient as an angry black man. Thanks to this insidious perception, Orville Blackwood paid the highest price possible.

The subtitle of the 1993 inquiry report was 'Big, Black and Dangerous?' Its eighty-seven pages told the story of a man who was trapped in a system that ultimately failed him.

Orville Blackwood came to London from Jamaica as a young child, ended up in care, then the mental health system and later

---

* There's a broader discussion here about whether schizophrenia should persist as a diagnostic label. Not all those who hear voices define themselves as having a disorder. Since there is no single genetic or pathological finding that explains schizophrenia, the term might, for now, be a placeholder, an umbrella term for a group of disorders yet to be understood or discovered, perhaps some with varying neurobiological explanations.

prison, initially for minor criminal offences. In the early 1980s, he developed auditory hallucinations and paranoid delusions. He was, at times, 'acutely disturbed', 'dishevelled', 'sexually disinhibited' and 'suspicious', according to his records from nine psychiatric admissions, most of them compulsory. His diagnoses were shifting – cannabis psychosis was an early one, later revised to schizophrenia. In 1986, he was sentenced to three years in prison after threatening staff at a bookmaker's with what turned out to be a replica gun. He remained at the specialist Broadmoor Hospital, sometimes in 'seclusion' – i.e. confined to a room he could not leave, isolated from other patients and constantly monitored – until his death, long after the end of his custodial sentence.

Although said to be popular with staff and patients, Blackwood was episodically paranoid and aggressive. His medication doses were escalated and it was felt that more staff were needed to restrain him over time. On 28 August 1991, he allegedly tried to punch a doctor (who had purportedly entered his room without warning). Blackwood was restrained by several nurses and received intramuscular injections of two major tranquilisers, one at three times the recommended dose, the other at twice the recommended dose. He was then left alone but 'almost at once, he stopped breathing'.

Orville Blackwood died in that seclusion room at the age of 31.

Two inquests recorded a verdict of accidental death and a coroner praised staff for their 'competence and attention to duty'. But Orville Blackwood was not the only black man to die in seclusion at the Broadmoor high-security facility – before him came Michael Martin and Joseph Watts. A 1993 inquiry was commissioned to investigate the circumstances of all three deaths. Its findings were damning. The subtitle of the report – 'Big, Black and Dangerous?' – drew on a phrase that staff at the hospital used openly. It encapsulated, the inquiry found, the misperceptions that drove staff behaviour and informed the circumstances of Blackwood's death.

There was no question that Blackwood had a long history of violent behaviour, but on the day of his death he had been resting quietly in his room. He had skipped lunch and then refused to go to occupational therapy. The inquiry criticised the 'provocative' decision of Blackwood's doctor to call for extra nurses 'to forcibly medicate a patient who was calm [...]. It seems not to have occurred to staff to ask [him] why he did not want to go'. It also highlighted the doctor's condescending use of the words 'my good sir' just before asking nursing staff to descend with injections.

There were institutionally biased practices at Broadmoor, the inquiry concluded. A knee-jerk response to any hint of resistance had developed – overuse of seclusion, high doses of antipsychotics, and restraint for black patients perceived to be hostile and confrontational. The mainly white staff at 'a white, middle-class institution in rural Berkshire' had 'little understanding of the needs and cultural differences of ethnic minority patients' and 'hyped up' the sense of danger patients posed. Devastatingly, the inquiry discovered that 'ethnic minority patients within the hospital are terrified that the authorities are "killing them off"', and cautioned that 'unless there is conscious effort to exclude the racist dimension in psychiatric care it is all too easy for psychiatrists and others to slip into the use of stereotypes, the "big, black and dangerous" syndrome'.

Perceptions at Broadmoor reflected those elsewhere. At the Maudsley in South London in the late 1980s, 50% of male African-Caribbean patients classified as non-violent were detained formally or in a locked ward, compared with 17% of white men. As for those deemed violent, the authors of one study stated that 'the Afro-Caribbeans tended to be younger, more verbally aggressive, more seriously violent and more psychotic. They are often big and physically strong. These are all factors which contribute to staff apprehension and to the use of restrictive measures'. In 1986, all West Indian patients at the Maudsley were detained in a locked ward at admission, compared with half of white men.*

This is not a problem of the past.

At one adolescent unit in South London between 2001–10, young black people with psychosis were around three times more likely than the White British group to have been detained. Asians in the same study were around twice as likely to be compulsorily detained.† This is a global issue and not simply due to a higher incidence of mental health disorders in these groups. A 2019 *Lancet* study of almost two million patients internationally (including Canada, Italy, Ireland, the Netherlands, US, Norway, Switzerland, Denmark, Spain and New Zealand) found that Black Caribbean and Black African patients were significantly more likely to be compulsorily admitted to hospital, compared with white ethnic groups – as were, to a lesser extent, south Asian patients. These disparities were most pronounced in the UK, where Black Caribbean and Black African groups also had more police contact and criminal justice involvement en route to psychiatric care. When Black Caribbean men and women are found by their GP to have a mental health issue, they are more likely to be referred to specialist mental health services than be looked after in primary care.

As we have seen, the cannabis psychosis and schizophrenia diagnoses, and their treatment, have embedded the perception of black men in particular as capable of great violence and hostility.

---

* The classification was based on the researchers' grouping of 'West Indian immigrants born in the Caribbean and British West Indians born in the United Kingdom'.

† 'Black' was defined as 'Black British', 'Black Caribbean', 'Black African' and 'Black Other'. 'Asian' included Indian, Pakistani, Bangladeshi and 'Asian Other'.

The consequence: greater levels of restraint, chemical suppression and seclusion. In 2011, the 23-year-old graduate student Olaseni Lewis was restrained by eleven police officers at Bethlem Royal Hospital in South East London. Lewis had no history of mental health issues, but had agreed to stay in the hospital overnight as a voluntary patient after his family noticed that he had become agitated. Lewis calmed down in hospital, but shortly after his family left for the evening at 8.30 p.m. he became agitated once again and tried to leave. A doctor called police to detain him under the Mental Health Act. Lewis was handcuffed, his legs were put in restraints, and he was struck with a baton. Another doctor later remembered the scene: 'I felt like it wasn't a human being that they were trying to restrain [...] after they had tied him up with the straps it seemed like when a hunter has tied the animal.'

Lewis lost consciousness and was taken to nearby Croydon University Hospital, where he was pronounced brain-dead. His life-support was turned off soon afterwards.

An inquest concluded that 'excessive force, pain compliance techniques and multiple mechanical restraints' used by police on Lewis had been 'disproportionate and unreasonable' and that 'on the balance of probability' this excessive force had contributed to his death. There were no criminal charges. Gross misconduct charges against six officers were dismissed, and three other officers left the force before disciplinary charges could be brought. One police officer had told the inquest that 'the sound and tone didn't suggest he had difficulty in breathing, more something on the inside of him, an aggression and a ferociousness that couldn't be controlled.'

A diagnosis medicalises a state and impels others to act on the assumptions that ensue. As the family of Olaseni Lewis discovered, sometimes those actions are carried out with fatal force.

Even now, in the 2020s, racialised diagnoses flourish, and increasingly it is children who are in the firing line.

The psychiatric diagnosis of oppositional defiant disorder (ODD) describes a hostile, vengeful, enraged and insolent child who develops behavioural problems, typically before the age of eight.* First listed as a psychiatric disorder in the 1980s by the APA, the term faced initial criticism for simply medicalising childhood temper tantrums and stubbornness, but with time the criteria have become refined, and ODD has increasingly become accepted internationally. Conduct disorders (ODD is included in this category in most UK studies) are now the most common mental health disorder in children and young people, and the most common reason in the UK for the referral of young children to mental health services. Up to one in eight children meets the diagnostic criteria for ODD at some point in childhood.

US studies show that the child diagnosed with ODD is usually black. Before puberty, ODD is more common in boys (this gender imbalance evens out later), which means that the archetypal younger child with ODD is a black boy: a seemingly angry, truculent and disruptive black boy. A parent who looks up their child's new diagnosis of ODD will see his future writ large: one commonly marked by an exit from the mainstream education system and entry into the criminal justice one. An educator who sees a child with ODD might lower their expectations and tighten their disciplinary procedures. The child, in turn, sees authority

---

* As per the official criteria published by the APA, the child with ODD shows a persistent pattern of angry or irritable mood, argumentative or defiant behaviour, and vindictiveness lasting at least six months. These behaviours are deemed significant enough to affect the patient's own functioning, and those around them. ODD is distinguished from other subtypes of conduct disorder by the extent and severity of antisocial behaviour.

figures lose hope and faith in him. He feels marginalised and alienated. Perhaps, without the support he needs, he steps away from the mainstream education system and, sometimes, towards the criminal justice one. His future has been foreshadowed by his diagnosis; he never has the chance to become anything else but the label he was given.

The overdiagnosis of ODD in black children, especially black boys, has parallels with the racialised diagnoses that have gone before it. When standardised child behaviour checklists are used to identify the condition in children with mental health issues, its prevalence reaches anywhere between 1% and 11%, and racial differences are largely absent. Yet real-world assessments tell a different story. When the medical records of community diagnosticians (making diagnoses based on their own judgement rather than standardised checklists) are analysed, racial disproportionalities are clearly evident even where behaviours between groups are similar: black children have an increased likelihood of being diagnosed with ODD when compared to white children. In some US studies, Latino youths have also been overrepresented.

Conversely, white children are more likely to be diagnosed with attention deficit hyperactivity disorder (ADHD) than black children. There is a striking distinction in how each diagnosis is approached. A diagnosis of ADHD is commonly perceived to be associated with biological factors and opens up the possibility of treatment with medications and behavioural therapy, and educational accommodation. In ODD, by contrast, defective parental behaviour is cited as a risk factor instead – textbooks routinely describe it as being grounded in family discord and harsh, neglectful or highly authoritarian parenting. Here, the treatment option is stark: 'parent management training'. The Parenting Program at UCLA, for instance, pledges to 'reduce yelling and arguing' in parents. It seems, then, that it's not only children with

ODD who are being judged and stigmatised, potentially for life, but their families too.

Ultimately, ODD leaves itself open to amplifying the false narrative of 'black and dangerous'. The potential bias, albeit sometimes unconscious and unintentional, of those who diagnose ODD informs their predictions that black children are less likely to meet mainstream expectations and more likely to exhibit dangerous behaviour.

UK research data on ODD is sparse, and tends to focus on the broader term of 'conduct disorder', but there are distinctions between these two diagnostic labels for disruptive behaviour, and it's unclear that research on one can be applied to the other. The clinical picture of conduct disorder is of someone who is hostile, vindictive, spiteful, argumentative and defiant. ODD is a condition of similar behavioural features, but is usually seen as a diagnosis for younger children who have issues with authority; while the child with conduct disorder, the criteria state, violates social norms and the rights of others, through physical aggression, property destruction, theft and bullying.

But even when studies in this country combine both diagnoses, the prevalence of conduct disorders is lower than average in children and young people of south Asian family origin, and higher than average in children and young people of African-Caribbean family origin. These differences are not explained by social disadvantage.

That ODD declares itself in childhood offers little protection. A US study showed that the perceived threat commonly associated with black men even seems to extend to black children as young as five. Black boys are seen as older than their white peers: when students (mainly white) were shown photographs of black, Latino and white boys, they overestimated the ages of the black boys (who were aged 10–17) by an average of four and a half years. A thirteen-year-old was viewed as an adult. In the same study, black boys were also seen as more culpable for their actions – innocence was not a quality afforded to them. As one of the researchers, Phillip Atiba Goff, later told the *Washington Post*, 'it's almost like childhood was invented to protect white boys only'.

In a chilling real-world parallel, in 2014 the same assumptions sealed the fate of twelve-year-old Tamir Rice in Cleveland, Ohio as he played with a toy gun. He was shot dead by a police officer who fired his gun within two seconds of getting out of his patrol car. An officer who later arrived on the scene stated 'the male looked to be 19 or 20 years old'.

The diagnosis of ODD was not designed with the intention to racially discriminate. It was conceived to distinguish which children with perceived oppositional behaviour and negativity lay 'outside the norm'. But psychiatric diagnoses, as we have seen with cannabis psychosis and schizophrenia, can be slippery and difficult to discern with certainty, and as such are acutely sensitive to the biases and beliefs operating around them.

The problem extends beyond the field of psychiatry, though. Diagnoses across the medical spectrum are vulnerable to un-adulterated explicit bias at an individual level, but also to implicit bias where those who make them live in a society shaped by wider cultural beliefs and stereotypes. Where black and brown bodies and minds are seen as 'other' and as lesser, the people who inhabit them are frequently forced to experience greater anguish from their first medical encounter. Minority patients are less likely to have their pain adequately treated, for instance. Even when their self-reports of pain echo those of white patients, they have a lower chance of receiving analgesia, and when they do receive it they are given lower doses. This is a pattern consistently seen for young black children with sickle cell anaemia and appendicitis. African American men presenting with chest pain at nationwide emergency rooms were up to 30% less likely to receive diagnostic tests such as cardiac monitoring or a chest X-ray. Unconscious stereotypes could contribute to this practice: half of more than 200 white medical students and residents in a 2016 University of Virginia study endorsed beliefs such as 'black people's skin is thicker than white people's skin' and 'blacks' nerve endings are less sensitive than [that of] whites'. These false beliefs, resolutely held despite their own medical training which comprehensively disproves them, fed into their assumptions – i.e. that black people feel less pain – and influenced theoretical treatment decisions: students who had endorsed these beliefs were less likely – at least hypothetically – to treat black people's pain adequately.

Diagnoses also exist in spaces where there is structural racism – defined as the social forces, institutions, ideologies and processes that interact with one another to generate and reinforce inequities among racial and ethnic groups. When we make a diagnosis of cannabis psychosis or schizophrenia we may seek information about our patients from their family or police officers or teachers, and those sources are susceptible to similar biases. These informants might see cannabis, for instance – or race or ethnicity – as relevant when they are not. They might draw upon misconceptions about genetic vulnerability and race and violence that they have absorbed, read or heard about before.

In October 1998, Jamaican-born David Bennett died at Norvic secure psychiatric unit in Norwich. The 38-year-old had initially been diagnosed with cannabis psychosis, and later with schizophrenia. He had been restrained face down for twenty-five minutes by up to five nurses. Six years later, an inquiry into his death labelled institutional racism a 'festering abscess' which remained 'a blot upon the good name of the NHS'. A number of moves to heal that abscess have proved to be less than a resounding success.* In 2018, Simon Wessely, a former president of the RCPsych, acknowledged that

> we have to accept [that] the painful reality of the impact of that combination of unconscious bias, structural and institutional racism, which is visible across society, also applies in mental health care. I know that many people will be made to feel uncomfortable by these terms; and indeed I was one of them.

A racialised diagnosis is born and empowered through systems that are institutionally racist.

These are the very spaces in which ODD, cannabis psychosis and schizophrenia operate – all carry connotations of violence and hostility. These diagnoses have been constructed and circulated in a time when even black *children* are seen as suspicious, as blameworthy, as other.

Diagnoses such as ODD and cannabis psychosis share an elusiveness of sorts; they deny simple characterisation, and the shadow they cast shifts in time and place and shape. They pose a danger to those who carry them. First, they attempt to distinguish behaviour that is abnormal – perceived to be unduly aggressive –

---

* Recent criticism of reports that aim to tackle mental health inequalities have highlighted that 'solutions' are targeted towards addressing individual bias ('cultural competency' training courses and the like) rather than broad structural and systemic factors. The views of those who have experienced structural racism, carers and communities are frequently undervalued and under-represented. Even within the medical workforce, BAME staff are under-represented at senior level and 15% have reported facing discrimination themselves.

by defining what is normal. And that is, by definition, a subjective task. Second, they do not possess a biological marker that asserts either presence or absence. A diagnosis does not need a single definitive biological marker to exist (otherwise we would have to reject anxiety and depression as diagnoses, for instance), but their absence in ODD and cannabis psychosis means that diagnosticians are reliant on checklists and interviews instead; and those are developed by medical professionals who are subject to biases and operating in structurally racist systems. The issue is not only one of misuse of a diagnostic label, but also inherently one of partiality in the very construction of the diagnosis.

It is true that these diagnoses are not necessarily designed with prejudicial ambitions, but some responsibility for the prejudicial consequences must be carried by those who construct the labels, disseminate and champion them. They exist in spaces where the diagnosed and their families have little opportunity to be heard.

These diagnoses will travel through clinics and hospitals and schools and police stations and prisons. They will change how the people so labelled are perceived and treated and punished, and sometimes killed. But it's not too late to change.

4

Ayesha's Escape

The orange buckets in this makeshift playroom are filled with gravel instead of sand. The crayon drawings are of mass graves and grenades, homes under attack and helicopters falling from the sky. In one, a family stands powerless as orange flames creep towards them, a little girl in a triangle-shaped skirt rooted to the ground, her tearful mother with a baby in a sling. It is signed 'Alex, aged 6'. Outside the tent, next to the vast Moria refugee camp near Mytilene on Lesbos, staff from MSF (Médecins Sans Frontières) hurry about, the static from their walkie-talkies punctuating the din of babies crying.

Ayesha is lying on a camp bed. She is nine years old. Her white T-shirt is emblazoned with a beaming koala. There are smaller versions of the koala on her white shorts. A pink headband sits atop straight auburn hair. As other children play hide and seek between tents, I am struck by her profound stillness; the only sign of movement is the rise and fall of her ribcage. There is life, I sense, but only in its most basic form.

Before the family left Afghanistan, Ayesha's father tells me, 'she was naughty and she was sweet. She played with dolls, she loved parks and sightseeing'. Now, a steel cage encircles her right leg, which was shattered in a suicide bomb attack. Pink ribbons on her sandals, scuffed nail polish, scarred feet. The blast killed her four-year-old brother.

Ayesha has survived a series of harrowing operations since the blast, and a trip across the sea to reach what her family had hoped would be the safety of Greece. Despite it all, Ayesha could still speak, could still smile, when she arrived here.

Then, two weeks ago, a teenager was stabbed to death close to her family's tent. 'There was blood and there were sirens,' her father tells me. 'Everyone was shouting. She started screaming. But then suddenly she had no words.' Since then, Ayesha has not opened her eyes or spoken. She has not stood or sat up. Her father feeds her a little mashed food each day, gently coaxing it into her mouth. It takes two hours to finish fifteen or so teaspoons.

Ayesha is not alone in entering this state of extreme withdrawal. It has been seen in other traumatised refugee and asylum-seeking children – there have been hundreds of recorded cases in Sweden, where it is called *Uppgivenhetssyndrom* ('resignation syndrome'), and some at Australia's offshore immigration detention centre on Nauru – but this is one of the first cases the medical team have seen at Moria.

I imagine the trauma declaring itself throughout the bodies of these children, regressing their minds and bodies with each twist and turn. They stop eating and drinking. Their muscles waste away. Their parents place them in nappies, in wheelchairs, learn how to hook them up to feeding tubes. The children linger in this state for months, even years, growing older yet ever less present. They only recover when – and if – their families find security and stability.

There is as yet no formal or widely accepted diagnosis for this state. Some medics describe it as a resignation syndrome, others as 'traumatic withdrawal syndrome' or 'traumatic refusal'. Formally, it is instead usually fitted into the broader and well-established diagnostic category of PTSD.

For now, Ayesha remains still, silent, perhaps too overwhelmed to contemplate her past, present, or future.

I have travelled to Lesbos to investigate the diagnosis of PTSD. I had little reason to question the utility of PTSD as a diagnostic label when I first encountered it as a doctor in Ireland and the UK, in survivors of car crashes or witnesses to violence. But my humanitarian work elsewhere – seeing how western experts hurry to conflict zones to champion imported treatments over indigenous expertise – has compelled me to interrogate whether the label of PTSD captures the experience of trauma solely through a western lens, ignoring the responsibility our nations should bear for the trauma we inflict on others. Yet there's another undeniable possibility: a diagnosis of PTSD could direct Ayesha towards treatment, and even lead her towards liberty. I hope that my time on Lesbos will help me understand where the truth lies.

I arrived in Mytilene as the sun rose over gleaming cruise ships and immense yachts and palm trees. Alongside the harbour were candy shops and boutiques – the sort that keep their doors shut even when they are open. Moria refugee camp, where I would meet Ayesha the next day, is a mere fifteen-minute drive from this well-heeled resort. The only sign of turmoil nearby was a discarded sign by a guesthouse: 'We take aid, not sides.'

At Mytilene's mental health clinic, run by MSF, shafts of light illuminate a sparse room. Haseeb, a seventeen-year-old shepherd boy, sits across from a psychiatrist, Maxine. When three of his friends were murdered by militia, Haseeb fled Afghanistan, arriving first in Iran, then in Turkey, before landing here. Flashbacks puncture his waking hours without warning, scattering like random gunfire. Relentless insomnia haunts his nights. But an insanity has arisen within him too. Sometimes, increasingly so these days, he sees people who don't exist, and hears voices that don't either. 'I see a figure in black but he has no face. He speaks, he is the one controlling me. Whatever he does, I do.' During these episodes,

Haseeb bites himself, tries to hang himself, jumps off ledges. Mercifully, he says, he remembers little of the episodes afterwards. Occasionally, glimpses return to Haseeb during therapy sessions. They do so today, as I am there with him – his distress fills the room.

In many ways, the diagnosis of PTSD speaks to Haseeb's experience. He has, of course, suffered trauma. He shares its other features listed in international classifications too – his re-experiencing of events through recurrent nightmares, and his intrusive, distressing memories. He is hypervigilant, he startles easily, he has angry outbursts.*

But there are things that don't fit. These psychotic hallucinations, this loss of grip on reality, have not typically been listed in the most widely used diagnostic criteria for PTSD.

The diagnosis of PTSD was not designed for Haseeb. It was conceived decades before, for groups of people who took a different journey from his: war veterans and assault victims and car crash survivors. I wonder if fundamental elements of Haseeb's experience might go overlooked and so go untreated, if he is forced to wear a diagnostic label that has been tailored to the needs of others.

Haseeb tells us that the figure he sees most days comes from

---

* According to the criteria in the fifth edition of the DSM, PTSD is characterised by a history of trauma exposure, and by four symptom clusters lasting more than one month, which cause significant distress or impairment in social, occupational or other important areas of functioning. The symptom clusters are: re-experiencing the traumatic event (for instance through intrusive, distressing memories, recurrent distressing dreams, or dissociative reactions such as flashbacks); avoiding anything that reminds one of the trauma, whether it be memories or conversations; clear changes in memory or mood; and alterations in physiological arousal and reactivity, such as angry outbursts and reckless behaviour, hypervigilance and exaggerated startle response.

outside his head, not inside it. It will return tomorrow, he is certain of it. He will be compelled to do what it says. Maxine puts down her pen, carefully puts aside Haseeb's ever-expanding file cataloguing his demons, looks into his eyes. 'I disagree,' she says. 'I think it's something your horrible memories have created. If it's true, what I'm saying, our job is to bring all the pieces together. Then there's not so much to be frightened of.'

Distress has been linked to traumatic events since antiquity. Although many descriptions in the sources that have come down to us are of short-lived grief, others align with today's definition of PTSD: intrusive, distressing memories and dreams, flashbacks, altered memories, low mood, anger, recklessness and hyper-vigilance.

When the Sumerian king Ur-Nammu (c. 2112–2094 BC) died in battle, anguish gripped his people: 'The people are seized with panic. Evil came upon Ur [...]. They weep bitter tears in their broad squares where merriment had reigned. With their bliss[fulness] having come to an end, the people do not sleep soundly.'

In August 1572, Charles IX of France described his torment in the aftermath of the St Bartholomew's Day massacre to his chief surgeon Ambroise Paré. He had ordered the killing of key Huguenot leaders in Paris, but the murders went far beyond those targeted in his plan; instead, Catholic soldiers and civilians carried out a widespread, relentless massacre, in defiance of Charles's royal orders to cease the killing. Thousands of French Protestants died across the country: 'I feel one in fever, my body and mind are both disturbed. Every moment, whether asleep or awake, sights of corpses, covered with blood, and dreadful to watch, haunt me. Oh, I wish they had spared the innocent and fools.'

It was not until centuries later that the psychological distress that can follow trauma began to be medicalised. This medicalisation did not materialise through some scientific breakthrough; no brain region was implicated in its anatomy, no protein identified in its pathology. Instead, the diagnosis of PTSD emerged in response to the Vietnam War. It was a political banner unfurled and a protest march recognised. It spurred on the granting of disability benefits and sympathy towards veterans of a war many could no longer believe in.

Before the Vietnam War, soldiers who experienced distressing nightmares and flashbacks, and sometimes physical symptoms like paralysis, blindness, palpitations or extreme fatigue, had been labelled with any number of syndromes: 'nostalgia' in Swiss mercenaries in the seventeenth to nineteenth centuries; 'soldier's heart' in the British army in the Crimea and in the American Civil War; 'shell shock' in the First World War; and 'combat fatigue' in US forces during the Korean War in the early 1950s.

Shell shock was often perceived as a sign of cowardice – especially if no courage had been shown before – as a character flaw, or as symptomatic of a personality trait. 'Artistic types', 'imaginative city dwellers' and the 'highly strung' were especially susceptible. Psychoanalytic theories linked the condition to 'inhibited libido' and a 'weakened sex drive'. It was even seen as potentially contagious to fellow soldiers. By the end of the First World War, 80,000 cases of it had been treated in Royal Army Medical Corps medical units, and 30,000 troops diagnosed with some form of 'nervous trauma' had been evacuated to British hospitals.

One sufferer of shell shock was Private Harry Farr, member of the 1st Battalion, West Yorkshire Regiment. Farr, who had been hospitalised for shell shock three times in 1915–16, refused one September morning to head to the trenches. The following morning, he was arrested and charged with contravening section 4(7) of the Army Act 1881 – showing cowardice in the face of the enemy. He was executed by firing squad. In all, more than 300 British and Commonwealth soldiers were executed during the First World War for cowardice or desertion.

The 1922 report by the War Office Committee of Enquiry into 'Shell-Shock' included a statement from Lieutenant-Colonel Viscount Gort, who said that shell-shock 'must be looked upon as a form of disgrace to the soldier'. The committee's final report was more benevolent, and acknowledged the 'true nature' of the condition. It ultimately recommended that the term 'shell-shock' be scrapped entirely. By 1930, the death penalty for cowardice in the military was abolished. It took until August 2006 for Harry Farr to be pardoned by the UK government, some ninety years after being sentenced to death.

As for the emergence of PTSD as a diagnostic label, it began with the return of Vietnam War veterans, who arrived home to find themselves under attack. 'Epithets like "babykiller" and "psychopath" were thrown at them by some enraged civilians,' writes psychiatrist Derek Summerfield. Initially diagnosed with a variety of ills – anxiety, personality disorders, schizophrenia, substance misuse – consolidation came when a section of the US anti-war movement, psychiatrists included, began to lobby the APA for a specific diagnosis that would allow specialised medical care for these veterans. 'Post-Vietnam syndrome' was forwarded for inclusion in DSM-III in 1980. 'The new diagnosis aimed to shift the focus of attention from the details of a soldier's background and psyche to the fundamentally traumatogenic nature of war,' Summerfield explains. 'Vietnam veterans were to be seen not as perpetrators or offenders but as people traumatised by roles thrust on them by the US military.'

Other groups advocated for their version of post-Vietnam syndrome too. An increasingly vocal anti-psychiatry movement was critical of speculative and stigmatising psychoanalytic models, which they believed drove pejorative attitudes towards child abuse survivors. A diagnosis of PTSD spoke to the broader influence of the malevolent forces that caused trauma, rather than the victim's supposed contribution to it.

This new entity of PTSD was introduced by DSM–III, published in 1980.* The diagnosis made room not only for veterans, but for anyone who showed significant distress in response to a 'stressor that would evoke significant symptoms of distress in almost everyone'. Nonetheless, it was the lobbying efforts of the Vietnam War veterans and their supporters that had brought PTSD into being as a label. According to Summerfield, it 'legitimised their "victimhood", gave them moral exculpation', while also bringing them a disability pension.

The diagnosis was soon extended to survivors of earthquakes and the frontline aid staff who came to their rescue; to witnesses of plane crashes and car pile-ups; to the incarcerated and injured. Each claim to its existence made at conferences and in compensation cases, in scholarly papers and self-help magazines, confirmed PTSD as a discrete entity. It set the scene for the founding of the International Society for Traumatic Stress Studies and the establishment of academic publications such as the *Journal of Traumatic Stress*. The WHO included the diagnosis in the ICD more than a decade after its first official appearance in DSM–III.

With each subsequent iteration of the DSM, the definition of PTSD shifted. Now the trauma is categorised as 'exposure to actual or threatened death, serious injury, or sexual violence'. Someone can suffer from PTSD after witnessing trauma as it

---

* The first edition of the DSM published in 1952 had acknowledged the possibility of 'gross stress reaction' resulting from 'combat or civilian catastrophe', but had removed this from the second edition.

occurs to others. As the definition has morphed, the number of diagnosed has spiralled.

The formulation of the PTSD diagnosis created a seismic shift in our perception of trauma and those whom it visited. Far from being confined to the cowardly and weak-willed soldier of old, the premise now was that anybody could suffer lasting distress in the face of trauma. Trauma itself – whether a sexual assault, a car crash or a bomb blast – was the defining moment, and sufficient. Oedipal fantasies, moral failings and sexual inadequacy did not need to be invoked. This new expression of psychological distress, now codified, did not insinuate malingering or monetary greed. Financial reparation instead became a legitimate response to it. Distrust and suspicion were no longer welcome. PTSD invited compassion where shell shock had frequently incited contempt. In *Empire of Trauma*, a tour-de-force exploration of how trauma has come to authenticate the suffering of victims, Didier Fassin and Richard Rechtman write: 'A century of clinical suspicion directed against traumatic neurosis patients by both civilian and military practitioners collapsed under the effect of this new definition'.

PTSD has informed our lives like few other psychiatric diagnoses. While some conditions described in the DSM are rarely used and others are primarily used for billing purposes or solely in academic circles (Avoidant Restrictive Food Intake Disorder is one such example), PTSD has established itself in our everyday vernacular.

Within twenty years of its birth, the diagnosis of PTSD had well and truly grown up. Not only that, it had gone travelling too. In June 2000, the *Lancet* published a paper from researchers in Freetown, Sierra Leone, a region that had seen sustained and intense violence. Of the respondents, 99% had scores 'that indicated very high levels of disturbances, indicative of severe PTSD'. In the study, PTSD was measured using a scale designed by psychiatrists at the University of California School of Medicine in San Francisco two decades before.

The diagnosis of PTSD had been exported.

Back at Mytilene's mental health clinic, Haseeb has left the room, taking with him his hallucinations of a faceless figure in black. He still fears that the figure will once again control his thoughts, his movements, his words, his future. Perhaps with time, that fear will fade a little.

I discover that specialists on Lesbos have seen many patients like Haseeb, who are not only haunted by flashbacks and angry outbursts and hypervigilance, all features of PTSD, but also by raging psychosis, seeing what others cannot see, hearing what others cannot hear.

Clare, a doctor who worked with trauma survivors for many years in her home country of Ireland before arriving here, says these patients on Lesbos present in a way she has never seen before. 'This is the first time I have seen psychotic symptoms – delusions, visual and auditory hallucinations [with trauma]. These people make contact with you in the room but they're seeing things like they're back in the Congo.'

The picture seemed so characteristic to psychiatrist Alessandro Barberio and his colleagues that they initially called it 'Lesbos syndrome', simply as a shared informal term of understanding at the camp. But then they realised they might be on to something. Case after case, all with the same constellation of symptoms – a seeming loss of the will to live and of their hold on reality. It usually occurred in young men, he realised, as the numbers rose. Sufferers would stop eating and washing and dressing. They would sit by their tents, silent, sorrowful, surviving only because fellow migrants, strangers often, tried to help them, feed them, sometimes coaxing them towards the clinic, by the hand, step by step.

One man who came to Alessandro's clinic had escaped from the militia in his home country. He was in his thirties, and was haunted by hallucinations when he reached the island. 'He was really anguished, his speech was slow, he made no eye contact,' Alessandro remembers. 'And each day, he would see in his mind his brother decapitated.' This wasn't a flashback, Alessandro told me; it wasn't a memory of an event that had happened. It was something that he felt was happening right there, right in front of him. Voices spoke to him: 'Don't get help, these people are useless, you will die'. Sometimes the voices spoke to one another, threatening, abusive. There were other visions too – the man would look down to find himself covered in blood, his hands soaked in it, his flesh putrefying, the smell permeating every pore.

Alessandro had heard of psychosis in traumatised refugees before, but it usually came about years after the initial trauma, once they had relocated permanently. On Lesbos, this psychosis was occurring soon after the refugees' arrival, while they were still in a state of limbo. There was another crucial difference, and this at least was a positive one – many patients in Moria responded within weeks to therapy and antipsychotic medications. The man who hallucinated beheadings and bloodshed quickly recovered with treatment. He was later reunited with the family whom he had feared dead.

Why, then, do Haseeb's and Ayesha's responses to trauma (his hallucinations, her resignation from the world) diverge so profoundly from those of the PTSD sufferer we usually hear about – the person who has been injured in a car crash or the soldier who returns from battle?

Perhaps their responses are different because the trauma is different. Haseeb's is not a single-incident trauma, a one-off like a traffic accident for example, as was envisaged by the early editions of the DSM. Instead, like many other refugees on Lesbos, he has been subjected to prolonged persecution, starvation, repeated assault, and ongoing uncertainty and stress. Some who are stranded in these camps suffered sexual violence or forced marriage in their countries of origin. They have seen loved ones tortured and murdered or disappeared.*

Maxine believes that the multiplicity of such traumas is relevant:

> I have worked in Zimbabwe, Liberia, Egypt, Bhutan
> and with American Indians, but this is a very specific
> situation because of trauma, because of loss of home and
> family. You've lost everything familiar to you, people
> who speak your language, your few possessions, you
> don't know what's in store for you when you leave.

For most of Maxine's patients, the journey to Lesbos has been perilous. They've faced exploitation along the way, been separated from their families, seen fellow migrants drown – thousands of them each year in the Mediterranean. Leema, our translator, tells me how the boat carrying her family almost sank during their crossing. Her six-year-old daughter watched the water as it rose. 'Can I eat the fish?' she asked. The family threw the clothes and scraps of food they had painstakingly stockpiled for their journey overboard. The island came towards them. When Leema placed her hand into the water, it was shallower than before. 'We will not die,' she told her husband, relieved. 'We will not die.' They reached land, but the memories of that near-drowning are etched into the fabric of her existence. She wonders if her children will carry the emotional scars forever.

---

* The most recent version of DSM-5 broadens its remit, noting that symptoms vary over time, with 'recurrence and intensification [...] in response to reminders of the original trauma, ongoing life stressors, or newly experienced traumatic events'.

On arrival, the refugees' struggle continues. On Lesbos, they face social isolation and discrimination. They have little access to food, shelter, money, familiar religious rituals and medical care. Some must live alongside the perpetrators of violence in their countries of origin. They are subjected to hostile government policies, extended detention and a convoluted asylum application process, with their human rights violated each day. We know that the resolution of someone's visa status plays a pivotal role in improved mental health. A mounting sense of injustice when perpetrators are not brought to account worsens it.

Separation from your family can also exacerbate mental distress. At Moria, I met sixteen-year-old Ahmed, who, like Ayesha, had no mental health problems before arriving on Lesbos five months earlier. Now his frequent and violent outbursts terrify those around him. 'Everything I see, everything I hear, the smallest things make me angry. A darkness comes over me,' he tells me. He cannot remember his brutality once the episodes fade. His mother, often the subject of his most vicious (and uncharacteristic) attacks, is with us today, trembling and broken. 'Have you harmed yourself?' the psychologist asks Ahmed. He pulls up his left sleeve – ragged scars criss-cross his forearm. He misses his little brother and his father, he says. He does not know where they are or whether his family will ever be reunited. Ahmed is not alone in his torment – in July and August that year, three children referred to the MSF clinics on Lesbos had tried to kill themselves and seventeen had self-harmed.

The features of psychosis experienced by Haseeb and Ayesha's withdrawal syndrome defy traditional definitions of PTSD. These symptoms of mental distress do not fit into the pre-ordained checklist that doctors use to diagnose the condition. Nor do the symptoms quite align with schizophrenia, depression or other recognised psychiatric disorders, Alessandro says.

Maxine is less interested in what we name it than she is in the question of how to best treat its sufferers. 'There is a constellation of symptoms following trauma here, call it what you want, I don't care about labels. We see withdrawal, mutism, hearing voices of persecution, insomnia. They wake up screaming, they have delusions that soldiers back home are coming after them.'

There is something that strikes me, in the stories I have heard. It is an obvious and yet brutal, devastating realisation: there is an unforgivable error at the heart of the PTSD diagnosis as it now exists. For Ayesha, for Haseeb, for Ahmed, there is no 'post' to their trauma. It is now, it is still happening. In these camps, they and many other refugees still suffer, still face inequity, still confront a system and society that wilfully ignores their plight.

Their trauma was yesterday, it is today, and it will inevitably be tomorrow.

Just as it seems impossible to capture the full spectrum of mental anguish within the diagnosis of PTSD, it is also a label that struggles to hold the complete, visceral picture of physical symptoms after trauma.

At the start of this book, we met Joyce. In a hospital in Beira, she told me of a range of symptoms – widespread pain, dizziness, and weakness in her arms and legs – for which blood tests and X-rays yielded no explanation. A local healer had declared her to be possessed by the spirits of soldiers who had fought in the civil war decades before. These sorts of corporeal symptoms in the aftermath of trauma are widespread in countries like Mozambique which have suffered bloody conflicts and political convulsions. Some Rwandan genocide survivors describe *ihahamuka,* a blockage of sorts of the lungs, where an overwhelming emotion stalls breath and obstructs words. Attending gacaca tribunals (a local justice system) often proves therapeutic. The anthropologist Christopher Taylor writes that there was something highly personalised about it:

Undoubtedly, Western medical nosology [disease
classification] would group the various symptoms
termed *ihahamuka* under the rubric of post-traumatic
stress disorder (PTSD), but this would obscure what
is Rwandan about it. In effect, the survivors were
somaticizing the experience of having endured extreme
terror, but they were doing so in a culturally specific way
related to their notions about the body.

In other words, the precise circumstances of those who manifest
ihahamuka (and it is not seen in all Rwandans) shaped their response
to trauma. Trauma declares itself in myriad ways, and it is influenced
just as much by where you are as what you have experienced.
Gastrointestinal distress, neck soreness, tinnitus and dizziness when
standing seemed to be a prominent response to trauma among some
Cambodian refugees. Senegalese refugees from the Casamance
region (held in refugee camps in the Gambia) commonly reported
increased body heat and general body pain, as did tortured Bhutanese
refugees. One group of Salvadoran refugees living in the north-
eastern US frequently described *el calor* – an intense heat which
rapidly pervaded the body, sometimes several times a day. Adelina
Valenzuela, a 56-year-old woman, likened it to a fire that spiralled
through her body and shot out of her, making her eyes bulge:

I felt like I was suffocating and that I was dying [and] I
went and turned on the cold water to take a cold shower
[…] the heat feels as if, you know, with a match [you
light] a sheet of paper and then swallow it, and inside the
heat that feels so terrible, those flames of fire welling up.

Somatic symptoms after trauma might be just as common in
western populations, but I sense that we often strive to label this

kind of suffering with a diagnosis that seems wholly 'physical', a condition indisputably rooted in the body. Numbness becomes carpal tunnel (even if the tests are borderline or exclude it); gastrointestinal distress is diagnosed as irritable bowel syndrome; dizziness is designated some form of vertigo, and so on. But perhaps, in reality, the expression of the traumatised patient's distress is no different from their counterpart in Beira.

In different cultures, then, we see different expressions of trauma, whether it's *ihahamuka* or *el calor*, and indeed the definition of PTSD has broadened over time, in an attempt to reflect trauma beyond a western lens. The APA acknowledges that 'clinical expression of symptoms [of PTSD] may vary cross-culturally with respect to avoidance and numbing symptoms, distressing dreams, and somatic symptoms'.

We can keep expanding the diagnosis of PTSD with Salva-doran heat and Cambodian dizziness and Haseeb's visions, but this constant expansion calls into question the diagnostic label in the first place. Already, there are almost endless permutations of symptoms that meet DSM criteria for PTSD, as captured by the title of one recent academic paper: '636,120 Ways to Have Posttraumatic Stress Disorder'.

PTSD is a diagnosis – a definition – in conflict. Over the decades, countless committees have gathered to broaden or narrow its criteria and description. They propose to use symptoms instead of clusters, to try more clusters rather than fewer, or add in putative and unproven biomarkers instead of bullet points. The WHO and APA carry different descriptions for PTSD, potentially leading to different prevalence rates depending on which system you use.

Trauma does not lend itself to neat classification. Although PTSD continues to be refined and redefined by consensus groups and workshops, an ever-expanding salmagundi of sorts, it strikes me that such an ephemeral constellation of symptoms cannot allow for definition at all.

The term 'PTSD' means little to Ayesha's father when he and I speak. He understands the power of a medical diagnosis, perhaps any diagnosis, in obtaining help for his daughter and escape for his family. But when I ask him how he would name his daughter's state, he hesitates. 'In my own language, we would call it brain damage, shock, fear,' he replies. There were idioms that the translator could not quite translate (and she was from the same city) – these expressions served him better than any equivalent English words could; this was a personal terminology that spoke to his own understanding of health and of his daughter's experience.

Perhaps one of the most serious accusations against the wholesale export of PTSD, and the one that underlies my gravest concerns about the diagnosis, is the suggestion that it functions as a tool of neo-colonialism. 'These concepts aggrandise the western agencies,' says Derek Summerfield, 'and their "experts" who from afar define the condition and bring the cure.' The privilege belongs to those who fly into the emergency zone, critics say, not those who are trapped within it. The empowerment is unilateral. Survivors with agency become submissive victims, usually treated by those self-appointed western 'experts'.

Programmes to address PTSD are promoted through humanitarian aid operations, at a cost of millions of dollars, and are enthusiastically backed by UNICEF, WHO and most nongovernmental organisations. The ethical concerns around conflict and political responses to it are muted in the process. Dispersing the label of PTSD across a conflict zone can mask the moral vacuum of war, conveniently reducing genocide to a series of diagnostic bullet points as it codes the casualties of battle. The diagnosis of PTSD even risks blame of sorts, or at least personal responsibility, being placed at the feet of trauma survivors. Recent guidance on mental health care from the WHO, co-published with the UNHCR (United Nations High Commissioner for Refugees), makes useful recommendations for strengthening social networks, but also advocates the provision of support to refugees so that they can 'identify and strengthen positive coping methods'. Why should recovery be predicated on individual fortitude when responsibility for that trauma extends far beyond one person?

Extended protocols encourage imported mental health teams to engage with local healers, religious leaders and anthropologists. The reality on the ground is revealed in one set of international guidelines, which suggests that 'healers may be prepared to learn how to monitor psychotic patients on long-term medication and to provide places for patients to stay while receiving conventional treatment.' According to this view, primacy is assigned to medicalisation and medication, and a label of PTSD – local healers are simply co-opted to carry out instructions.

In Joyce's case, harnessing healers to supervise and deliver westernised psychiatric treatment might have ignored the root causes of her distress, undermined local understanding of spirit possession, and denied her and her family the healing ceremony they were instead able to experience.

The danger of ignoring local customs and expertise is evident from the experiences of Mozambican refugees living in the borderland of Malawi's Dedza district and Mozambique's Angónia district, where talking therapy – a western approach to treating PTSD – was explored as a treatment option. But research conducted by the anthropologist Harri Englund during this time – in the early 1990s – found that remembering traumatic experiences could potentially be harmful. This community (mostly Catholic and from the Ngoni ethnic group) conceived of funerals as a time of remembrance, but also ultimately of forgetting: throwing soil into the grave (*kuponya dothi*) was said to help the bereaved not to think (*kuganizira*) about the deceased, to erase the presence of the deceased from their consciousness. After this step, it was 'no longer appropriate to reminisce about the deceased'. Western counselling methods posed a serious threat: 'The dead occupy an afterworld, and crucial to the separation of the two worlds are the attempts of the living to erase their personal memories of the dead. In such a context, the therapist's desire to make refugees talk about their dead relatives is likely to aggravate refugees' plight.'

The bereaved were primarily distressed because the graveyards for their loved ones were far away in Mozambique – to bury the deceased in their own villages, a long-standing tradition, had become an impossible feat. To compound the situation, the food aid they received at the camp lacked provisions for funeral guests or vengeful spirits. Instead of diagnosing PTSD and funding expensive individual counselling, humanitarian organisations would do better, Englund wrote, to support refugees in properly burying and mourning their dead. What they would value most, he wrote, was simple assistance in obtaining the materials they needed for burial: timber and cloth for a coffin. Perhaps, though, one of the greatest dangers posed by these experts flying in from afar is not necessarily the application of a diagnosis, if one is even warranted in the first place, but instead the assumption that healing can only be found in tablets and western therapy. This approach overlooks the importance of fostering extended support systems – it undervalues the strongholds and safe havens provided by family and social bonds, by economic and political stability. This 'tablets and therapy' strategy can represent a flawed philosophy not just in the approach to PTSD in conflict zones, but closer to home too.

The neo-colonialism argument is, to my mind, a compelling one, but it risks eroding the agency and resilience of the diagnosed. It may also do a disservice to the ambitions of early humanitarian missions that addressed psychological suffering, for example during the 1988 Armenian earthquake. These were not driven by any knowledge of, or by the practices that arose from, the new definition of PTSD. The initiator of MSF's psychiatric programmes recalled that 'our intervention wasn't based on that diagnosis. All the links to it were made after the fact, but they're of no historical value since we weren't thinking along those lines at all.' Instead, psychologists and psychiatrists simply strived to identify and care for those experiencing distress. Clearer evidence of humanitarian psychiatry starting to draw on the language of PTSD emerged during the 1990s in the former Yugoslavia, as missions entered Croatia, Bosnia and Kosovo.

The use of that language gradually spread, and today it forms the keystone of humanitarian practice in many regions. It lives on here in Moria and in the work of Alessandro, Maxine and the other humanitarian workers. The label of PTSD should never define sufferers entirely, or take absolute precedence over traditional customs and cultural understanding – but equally, to dismiss the diagnosis entirely may do a great injustice to Ayesha and the other traumatised children I've met on the island.

When I first went to Lesbos, I had come across many critiques of the diagnosis of PTSD arguing that it assumes a line inevitably leading from trauma to troubled mental health in the medium or long term; that it insists that the emotional responses arising in the aftermath of trauma are pathological and problematic. These are reasonable criticisms – sometimes a psychological reaction to trauma, as distressing as it might be, is part of a normal, adaptive human response. But these arguments about the over-medicalisation of distress are often thrashed out at length in academic papers and by think tanks, far removed from the reality of what is happening in refugee camps and conflict zones.

Our emotional existence – our lived experience – is fluid and dynamic and personal. How can a psychiatric diagnosis possibly capture its subtleties? The diagnosis of PTSD, despite its shortcomings, allows clinicians quickly to identify groups of people suffering distress in the aftermath of conflict, even in those believed to have 'inherited' a trauma that has been handed down through generations, for example in the case of Holocaust survivors. In Northern Ireland, where suicide rates are among the highest in the world (rates doubled in the ten years following the 1998 peace agreement), identifying those with a high suicide risk is crucial in helping them before it's too late.* But how to do that? One way is to use a diagnosis like PTSD, screen patients for the condition using its criteria, as fallible as they may be, and then offer mental health support to those who appear to be suffering most severely. Identifying these sorts of patients and patterns can allow advocates to push for resources where they're needed most.

Without exception, every ardent PTSD critic I spoke to on the ground ultimately acknowledged that the diagnosis has its uses. As one psychologist on Lesbos told me, 'PTSD is useful as a shared language since people in the hospital and on the mainland know what we are talking about – they know these children have experienced trauma and they are suffering.' A diagnosis can be used as evidence of human rights violations or as the cornerstone for an application for asylum. It will be, perhaps, a passport to the mainland for Ayesha. It speaks to her vulnerability, it directs her towards care, and, we must hope, towards compassion. Her trauma, a stamped document will imply, is legitimate because her doctors say so. It is counted, it is acknowledged. She is counted, she is acknowledged.

---

* In a recent World Mental Health Survey, Northern Ireland was found to have the highest level of PTSD (12-month and lifetime rates) among more than 30 countries.

The diagnosis of PTSD stands as shorthand for 'remove me from this place', 'hear my asylum plea', 'acknowledge my distress', 'provide me with the tools to heal'. In this, it has undeniable utility.

Later that month, I travelled to Athens to meet men and women who gained asylum and found safe harbour. They told me that they drew on the term 'PTSD' to agitate for change for other trauma survivors – PTSD is a diagnosis understood by disparate audiences across the political divide. It has allowed them to navigate bureaucratic systems and access legal assistance – who are we, then, to deny them the utility, the necessity, of a diagnostic label?

Some weeks after I first saw Ayesha, she was sent to the mainland for a specialist clinic appointment. The doctors there tried a medication that is normally used for anxiety, but she didn't respond to it. Last time I heard, the family had been returned to Moria and were still waiting to hear the outcome of their asylum application. Ayesha was not speaking or walking, and was barely eating. A psychologist told me she held out hope that Ayesha might receive a blue stamp on the basis of her diagnosis – an official certification of her PTSD that would improve the family's chance of being moved to the mainland.

The diagnosis of PTSD is an imperfect one. But I must acknowledge that my misgivings about it before I reached Lesbos were misplaced. They seem academic now. The diagnosis of PTSD need not define Ayesha, but it may be the only one that recognises her past and opens the door to a better future.

5

Behind Police Lines

On the autumn day in 2003 when he died at Thornhill police station in Birmingham, Mikey Powell, a father of three, was thirty-eight years old. A few weeks after his death, five hundred people marched here in his memory. They faced off against riot police behind a metal barrier. The demonstrators held placards saying 'We remember Mikey Powell', and 'Another death in police custody'.

When a judge later reviewed the CCTV footage from the station, he disallowed it as evidence because of the poor audio quality. As Mikey's body lay motionless in a cell, a film called *The Dogs of War* was playing in the custody suite. It was impossible to disentangle the conversations and the commotion that arose once Mikey was found in his cell dying, perhaps already dead, from the soundtrack of the war film, with its screaming, submachine guns and helicopters.

Mikey's death was blamed on a condition called 'excited delirium'.

We have already begun to see how diagnostic labels are influenced and informed by forces and stakeholders far from the medical front line. Through Mikey Powell's story, we now observe those stakeholders enter the research laboratory, the emergency room and, with tragic inevitability, the autopsy suite. Critics of the diagnosis of excited delirium claim that external stakeholders are using the diagnosis to distract from – or even conceal the use of – inappropriate restraint and unlawful force.

To investigate this contentious diagnosis, I return to the events of September 2003, when Mikey Powell's mother called the police, asking them to help her son.

It wasn't the first time Mikey had encountered the police. Several years before, 'Mikey went up onto the roof of an adjoining building to his mother's; it was a small building, two storeys with a flat roof,' remembers his cousin Tippa. Mikey's mother, Claris, called the police, who spent two hours with him and talked him down. 'Then she gave him a cup of tea, the police had a bit of banter with Mikey and they left.'

After this incident, Mikey went back to his normal life. 'He was very well known in the local area and he put on blues parties and late-night reggae parties in people's houses,' Tippa tells me. 'He was a normal run-of-the-mill guy, really, a fun-loving dad, a really dedicated dad. He looked after his mum, spent half his time at hers, and the other half with his partner and kids.'

Mikey had experienced mental health issues intermittently over the years, but had managed well on medications from his family doctor. He had a full-time job at a metal factory in Birmingham. When the company downsized, they kept him on. 'They knew about his mental health issues,' Tippa says, 'but they made allowances for the days when he felt unwell, he could make up the time later. They kept him on because he was a committed worker, he was always on time.'

On 7 September 2003, Mikey experienced a psychotic episode, this time smashing the window of his car and a window at his mother's house. 'My aunty was a typical Caribbean person of that age who views people in uniform with respect,' says Tippa, 'and because of that first experience she called them again the second time it happened. She thought they would just talk him down.'

When the police arrived, two officers shouted at Mikey to get down on the ground. Mikey took off his belt and hit their car with it. The police drove at him and ran him down. The officers sprayed him with CS gas, struck him with a baton and handcuffed him. Several other officers arrived and he was restrained by up to eight of them for more than fifteen minutes.

'His mother was pleading with the police to take him to a place of safety, to hospital, where he could be treated. He was injured from putting his hand through the police patrol car window, he was injured from the police car [hitting him].'

Instead, Mikey was taken to Thornhill Road police station: 'A minibus came and they wedged him in the aisle between seats for the whole journey with officers kneeling on his back holding down his legs and arms in a prone position that made breathing difficult,' Tippa says.

At the station, he was carried into a cell. At this point, the officers realised that Mikey had stopped breathing.

Ten officers were later charged with criminal offences, ranging from dangerous driving to assault and misconduct in public office. But their defence team argued that a medical condition might have caused Mikey's death. That condition was excited delirium, which had been described in a small number of textbooks and academic and legal papers, but not recorded in most international diagnostic classification systems, including that of the WHO.

Excited delirium is a state characterised by rapid breathing, profuse sweating, superhuman strength and stamina, and elevated body temperature. Its other criteria, primarily developed by medical examiners with input from law enforcement officials, include physically struggling with law enforcement or a failure to respond to police presence. Its physical symptoms are perhaps all equally applicable to a petrified person frantically battling to escape brutal force.

In the end, the Crown Prosecution Service's case was hampered by the poor quality of CCTV footage at the police station where Mikey Powell died. All the officers were acquitted. No disciplinary charges were brought.

Tippa has little time for the idea of excited delirium. 'It's bogus. It seems to be a tool used to shift blame off officers to the person who was restrained,' he says. 'You take Mikey, they said the way he was behaving, he was showing the classic signs of excited delirium. He wasn't. He was having a psychotic episode. There were ways to deal with that. You don't relabel it simply to explain away his death.'

An inquest into Mikey's death took place in 2009. The jury determined that, on the balance of probabilities, Mikey had died from positional asphyxia following police restraint. The pathologist Jack Crane concluded that a 'critical' event had happened during Mikey's transport to the police station. Forcing an exhausted person to lie on their front with their hands handcuffed behind their back 'is one of the most dangerous positions an individual can be put in. We have a person fully conscious when put in the van. A short time later he's effectively dead and suffers a cardiac arrest'.

In September 2013, a decade after Mikey Powell's death, West Midlands Police denied liability but apologised for the pain and suffering caused to Mikey's family. At the time, another cousin of Mikey's – the poet, novelist and playwright Benjamin Zephaniah – said the apology was better than nothing:

'But it's only a little bit better than nothing. What is important is that we let it be known that although we accept this apology, we are intelligent enough to know that it is just an apology. It is not justice.'

Mikey's mother has never really recovered, says Tippa. 'It had a massive impact, because she called the police, and to this day she blames herself.'

★

Excited delirium is an international syndrome, cited since 1985 in academic and media reports in Japan, Canada, Australia, New Zealand, Malaysia, South Africa, Switzerland, Ireland, Spain, Poland, Sweden, Iceland, Slovakia and the Netherlands, among others.

In the UK, excited delirium has been cited, mostly uncontested, in up to two dozen deaths since 1996. It is most frequently diagnosed in black and ethnic minority groups, and those with substance use and mental health issues. In recent years, a related syndrome called acute behavioural disturbance or ABD (which includes the state of excited delirium) has also been cited multiple times in the deaths of those restrained by law enforcement. Its 2019 inclusion in official guidelines from the Royal College of Emergency Medicine (RCEM) means that number is set to rise significantly.

In the US, the label of excited delirium has been cited in hundreds, perhaps thousands, of deaths to date. Some estimates stand at around 800 cases a year. In Texas alone, excited delirium was cited in at least 50 custodial deaths between 2005 and 2016, and in Florida, it appeared in 85 autopsy reports between 2009 and 2019. Both of these numbers are thought to be conservative estimates, since the label is not always made public unless a case goes to court. Nobody is keeping count of the numbers nationwide.

So how did excited delirium come to be? Long before it arrived in the UK and the Birmingham courts, it was drawn in the chalk outlines surrounding the bodies of 32 women across Dade County, Miami. Throughout the 1980s, they had been found dead in alleyways and stairwells and motels and parking lots across the city. Autopsies 'conclusively showed that these women were not murdered', Dr Charles Wetli, a coroner and professor at the University of Miami, told the *Miami News* in 1988. Instead, these women's deaths bore the hallmarks of a syndrome he had seen several years before, one related to chronic cocaine use in men and affecting the brain's nerve receptors. These drug users, Wetli claimed, had attained superhuman strength in their dying moments. They were unhinged and paranoid. One 26-year-old man stripped naked and smashed up his apartment. Another ran down the street screaming, then stole and fired an officer's gun. Cocaine was to blame, wrote Wetli and his co-author, the psychiatrist David Fishbain, in a 1985 paper entitled 'Cocaine-induced Psychosis and Sudden Death in Recreational Cocaine Users' published in the *Journal of Forensic Sciences*. But perhaps all was not as it seemed. Blood concentrations of cocaine were about ten times lower in these cases than would usually be seen in fatal overdoses; and all of the men diagnosed had died after being restrained, many within just a few minutes of police confrontation.

The 32 dead women from Dade County had suffered from the very same syndrome, Wetli believed, as the men who had seemingly lost their minds on drugs. The women were described in media reports as 'prostitutes' and 'crack cocaine addicts'. Almost all were black. Police reports suggested that all had had sex in the hours before their demise, and had used drugs. There were salacious details of their deaths in the media, but little about their lives:

'For some reason,' said Wetli – deputy chief medical examiner for Dade County at the time – 'the male of the species becomes psychotic [after chronic cocaine use] and the female of the species dies in relation to sex.'

Linda Johnson was found on 9 August 1988 in a field behind a school, lying beneath pine trees. 'At the head is a plain pink tanktop with blue letters spelling "Body Shop". Above her head are pink pants that are inside out. No other clothing anywhere at the scene [...]. [There] are electric cords also hanging from [...] the tree and these are consistent with ligatures'.

Barbara Black was found in a yard on 4 October 1988, a turquoise tube top pulled down about her trunk, 'otherwise nude'.

Barbara Lattimore, found by a drive-in cinema on 27 October 1988, 'partially nude, had a pink blouse pulled over [her] breast along with a white bra, her blue jeans were off but still on her left ankle [...] her eyes were clear'.

Brenda Hernandez was found in an open field on 4 April 1989; the medical examiner's report said she was barefoot, dressed in a 'pullover smock', 'nude from the waist down [...] the bra is partially pulled up [...] abraided marks present adjacent to her neck'.

The deaths of these Miami women could be explained away by a syndrome Wetli first called 'neural exhaustion' and later excited delirium. What bolstered his theory was the assumption that these 32 women had taken drugs too.

Lynette, a sex worker along Biscayne Boulevard who spoke to the *Los Angeles Times* in May 1989, had little time for these theories of neural exhaustion. 'A bad dude is taking out the girls,' she said. 'Of course, we're just a bunch of black whores. He'd go do it to a white woman and you'd see the FBI, the CIA and the Marines down here, for a thing like this.'

It wasn't long before Wetli's sex-and-drugs theory fell apart. An autopsy confirmed that one of the victims, fourteen-year-old Antoinette Burns, had died without any cocaine in her system. A medical examiner reviewed findings from thirteen of the dead women and found bruises on their necks, bite marks and signs of asphyxiation. They had been murdered.

In 1989, police identified the convicted rapist Charles Henry Williams as their prime suspect. One of the victims, nineteen-year-old Patricia Johnson, had a bite mark on her breast that matched Williams's dental records, and semen at the murder scene also matched his. Although the 37-year-old denied having sex with Johnson, he did concede to having sex with some of the other murdered women in their final hours. Police also had accounts from women who had escaped from him, and witnesses confirmed they saw him with six of the victims. Williams was already serving a forty-year prison term for rape, with seven previous arrests for the same crime (he was successfully convicted of three of them). He died in 2005 of an AIDS-related illness, before he could face trial.

By the time of Johnson's death, Wetli had turned to private practice. He had not discarded his hypothesis: 'The guy never went to trial, so we'll never know. The police had a commendable theory in suspecting him. But believing in something, and proving it, is another story.'

The syndrome of excited delirium, which had its origins in the cocaine- and sex-induced psychosis that Wetli had described, quickly made its mark. It was mentioned in case studies that featured in scholarly papers and conference proceedings in the 1980s and 1990s, assisted by reports from the very officers who had restrained the victims (almost invariably men) in their final moments. The definition of the condition was refined in each publication that supported the diagnosis, soon backed by a position paper from the US National Association of Medical Examiners (NAME) – the professional organisation for officials who determine cause of death, including deaths that are suspicious or sudden, or thought to be unnatural or unexplained. Later, the American College of Emergency Physicians (ACEP) also got on board, formally stating in an influential white paper:

'It is the consensus of the Task Force that ExDS [excited delirium syndrome] is a unique syndrome which may be identified by the presence of a distinctive group of clinical and behavioral characteristics that can be recognized in the pre-mortem state.'

In almost every case of excited delirium, these publications agreed, cardiac arrest and death occurred within minutes of cessation of a violent struggle. The characteristics listed in their criteria were alien to any previous diagnostic label: being naked or 'inappropriately clothed' was one feature of the diagnosis, as was exhibiting an 'attraction to or destruction of glass and reflective surfaces'. These victims were described as 'irrational and physically resistive', 'lacking remorse or normal fear' and 'making unintelligible animal-like noises'.

The diagnosis not only implied that the victim had accelerated their own death; it seemed to exonerate those around them. The ACEP stated that 'an elevated temperature may suggest that a life-threatening disease or condition was present, and that the death was independent of the police intervention'.

Excited delirium was often described as a syndrome (a collection of signs and symptoms, thought to be characteristic of a condition) rather than a disease (a malfunction in our physical or psychological processes – a condition whose cause appears to be clear). As a result, any number of symptoms in constellation could easily tick perhaps not quite all the boxes, but – conveniently – just enough of them to make the label stick.

In 2003, the *Los Angeles Times* reported that by some estimates excited delirium was now being identified as the reason behind the majority of all in-custody deaths. San Francisco's assistant medical examiner described it as a spiralling epidemic: 'This is happening every day. Every time you hear of a man acting crazy and running naked in the middle of the street or someone on drugs comes into the emergency room with six police officers on their arms, it's excited delirium.'

Soon, excited delirium reached reality TV. 'Help. Officers. Air! Help! Up! Oh God. Oh God. Oh God. You're killing me!' cried Donald Lewis in 2005, as the camera crew of *Cops* filmed some of his last words while police wrestled him to the ground, binding his arms and legs behind him. The Palm Beach medical examiner concluded that Lewis had died because of 'sudden respiratory arrest following physical struggling [during] restraint due to cocaine-induced excited delirium'. This death could not, the implication was, represent an abuse of police power. It was instead attributable to an abuse of drugs. A subsequent lawsuit citing the use of excessive force saw Michael Baden, a former New York City chief medical examiner, testify that Donald Lewis had actually died of asphyxia caused by neck compression. That lawsuit was later dismissed by the Supreme Court.

'I can't breathe,' they gasp in their final moments. 'Help' and 'please' and 'sorry'. These are the words I hear in the inquest footage I watch of men with knees on their necks or their faces pressed to the ground. They are the last words before silence descends. Blue uniforms above them, bloodstained pavement beneath.

A recurring theme in these deaths is the use of excessive and forceful restraint. Positional asphyxia, cited as the probable cause of death at Mikey Powell's inquest, occurs when someone is placed in a position that prevents or impedes normal breathing. It has been implicated in at least 26 of 38 restraint-related UK deaths over the past decade.

One of those deaths was that of Terrence Smith in Surrey, in November 2013. His family had called for medical help when Smith, aged thirty-two, became increasingly paranoid, distressed and agitated at home. He had taken amphetamines at some point beforehand, ran outside in his underwear and shouted at the sky. When paramedics arrived, they called for police support. Smith was handcuffed and put in leg restraints and a spit hood (which can impede breathing) and later a body cuff which took twenty-five minutes to apply. CCTV footage taken in his cell showed Smith gasping 'I can't breathe' thirteen times, and 'I can't take the pain no more'. He subsequently had a cardiac arrest and died in hospital the following day. Excited delirium was cited as a cause of death. Afterwards, Smith's family said:

> Instead of treating him as a patient, the police treated him like a criminal. The manner in which he was restrained was barbaric. The type and nature of the restraint, and in particular the use of the spit hood, was beyond anything we expect to see in a civilised society.

At the inquest into Terrence Smith's death, police officers were found to have used 'prolonged and excessive restraint'. There was, a coroner concluded, 'a failure to understand that the resistance to the restraint was leading to an ongoing depletion of oxygen and an increased level of adrenaline'.

Restraint was identified as the cause of death in post-mortems of 10% of police custody deaths between 2004 and 2015 in England and Wales.* Between April 2020 and March 2021 alone, there were 19 deaths in or following police custody. Twelve of the nineteen people who died were physically restrained, either by police officers or by members of the public (only one restraint-related death solely involved a member of the public, however).† The Independent Office for Police Conduct (IOPC) report on these cases emphasises that 'the use of restraint, or other types of force, did not necessarily contribute to the deaths'. Countless

---

* The eight prosecutions of police officers in connection with a death in custody (not all restraint-related) of the last fifteen years have all ended with acquittals – including prosecutions for murder and manslaughter – despite several unlawful killing verdicts in coroners' inquests.

† These figures from the IOPC do not include deaths related to police restraint in mental health settings – for instance, when officers are called in to help medical staff who are dealing with a patient not under arrest.

independent inquiries into restraint-related deaths in UK custody have emphasised the need to prioritise de-escalation (persuasion, calming techniques and negotiation), and yet the deaths continue to occur.

But there's one other factor I want to highlight about deaths for which excited delirium is cited. When we talk about restraint, we also need to consider the question of who it is used against. Even though black and minority ethnic deaths in police custody in England and Wales are proportional to other communities overall, the proportion of those deaths in custody that feature restraint is more than twice that of other deaths in custody. Black and minority ethnic men are more likely to die in restraint: Sean Rigg, aged forty, died at Brixton police station in 2008. Four years later, an inquest jury found that 'the level of force used on Sean Rigg whilst he was restrained in the prone position for eight minutes at the Weir Estate was unsuitable'. Leon Briggs, aged thirty-nine, died in Luton, after being restrained for more than 13 minutes, calling out 'please help me' before he died. Kevin Clarke, aged thirty-five, died after being restrained for 33 minutes by up to nine officers in Catford in 2018. Police body-cam footage shows Clarke repeatedly telling them 'I can't breathe' and 'I'm going to die'. In a narrative verdict, an inquest jury found that restraint 'probably more than minimally or trivially' contributed to his death. This pattern of racial disparity is echoed elsewhere in the world. In Minneapolis, for example, where George Floyd died in 2020 while an officer pressed a knee into his neck for at least 8 minutes and 15 seconds, police officers 'used force against black people at a rate at least seven times that of white people' between 2015 and 2020 (an officer at the scene said, as Floyd lay dying, 'I am concerned about excited delirium or whatever'). The American Civil Liberties Union states that the label of excited delirium is a means of 'whitewashing' excessive use of force, and notes that most reported cases involve black men.

The danger of an excited delirium diagnosis is that it diverts attention from the true causes of death, that is, complications arising from restraint and asphyxia. It clouds our perception of the chain of events that have led to someone's death, perhaps it even conceals them. The story of Robert Dziekanski shows just how easily this can happen.

In October 2007, a forty-year-old man left Poland and flew to Vancouver to join his mother, who had moved to Canada a few years earlier. Robert Dziekanski, a typesetter and later a tradesman, had a love for geography. He had bought atlases of Canada in preparation for his new life in 'the land of milk and honey'. But although the maps he owned – he was a collector – spanned the globe, Dziekanski's fear of flying had prevented him from ever visiting these far-flung places. He had never been on a plane. In the weeks before his trip, he grew increasingly anxious. He had a panic attack at his home in Gliwice just as he was due to leave – his friends described him as 'shaky', clinging to a radiator in his apartment. He had not slept for forty-eight hours. He was, however, calm by the time he boarded his flight. Having landed at Vancouver International Airport and successfully cleared the line for the Primary Inspection Kiosk, he became confused about how to proceed to Secondary Customs and Secondary Immigration. He spoke Polish and Russian, but no English.

I watch CCTV footage of his next few hours – his last. He is wearing grey trousers and a white jacket, and pulling a small black suitcase behind him. Walking back and forth, alone, he misses the entrance for Secondary Customs. Outside, his mother has arrived at the airport, but she cannot find her son. The hours pass and she frantically seeks information from a 'visitor information counsellor', customer service agents and Border Services officers. Almost nine hours later, she is told by a Border Services officer (who searched the Secondary Immigration area but not the entire customs hall) that there is no sign of her son and she might as well go home, since he must not have boarded the flight in the first place. The officer does not check the computer system to confirm Dziekanski's arrival. His mother, an office cleaner, drives the 370 km home, planning to return the next day.

Meanwhile, the CCTV footage shows that Dziekanski has finally been helped by a different Border Services officer through Secondary Customs and onwards to Secondary Immigration. Later, officers reported that he was thirsty and 'visibly fatigued'. They try to contact his mother – paging her, searching for her in the meeting area, eventually leaving a voicemail on her home phone. They approve Dziekanski's application for immigration and congratulate him on becoming a landed immigrant. He is escorted to the semi-secure International Reception Lounge. He wishes the officer goodnight and says 'thank you' in Polish.

Soon after, he becomes increasingly agitated and disorientated. He does not know where his mother is. It is 12.40 a.m.; he arrived in Vancouver at 3.15 p.m. Witnesses describe his behaviour as upset, nervous, distraught and bizarre. He is sweating, breathing heavily, and appears to be talking to himself. He throws a computer to the floor. He uses suitcases and a chair to form a barricade around himself. Next, the footage shows him throwing a small table to the ground behind a plexiglas screen. Nobody is in danger. The security guard and the other travellers are on the other side of the screen. None of the witnesses interviewed during the subsequent investigation felt threatened by Dziekanski. I hear someone on the video say to the security officer, 'He's so scared, just leave him.' Another passenger approaches him to offer help. Next, four officers from the Royal Canadian Mounted Police arrive. It is now 1.28 a.m. Dziekanski remains calm and cooperative, with his hands at his side. However, surrounded by the four officers, he soon becomes frustrated. 'Leave me alone. Have you lost your minds? Why?' he asks in Polish.

He is not aggressive, however. As Justice Thomas R. Braidwood later noted in his inquiry:

> I do not believe that either of these officers honestly perceived that Mr. Dziekanski was intending to attack them or the other officers. Neither officer carried out an appropriate reassessment of risk immediately before deployment of the weapon. They approached the incident as though responding to a barroom brawl and failed to shift gears when they realized that they were dealing with an obviously distraught traveller.

Within 6 seconds of asking police if they had lost their minds, Dziekanski has been tasered in the chest. I see him stumble to the right and fall to the floor, screaming, distraught. He is writhing around on the floor, kicking his legs. One second later, the taser is deployed again by the same officer. Now Dziekanski's body slightly curls up. He continues to scream, his arms raised into his chest and fists clenched, his legs cycling around helplessly. The officers move in and handcuff him. One places his knee with some force on Dziekanski's neck. Dziekanski is tasered again. Within ten seconds of being handcuffed, his breathing becomes laboured. Now he lies motionless.

Dziekanski does not receive CPR until paramedics arrive on the scene fifteen minutes later. They find him still handcuffed, his face blue, his lips and tongue similarly cyanotic. He is not breathing, and he has no pulse. He is pronounced dead after twenty minutes of CPR.

Several experts cited excited delirium at the inquiry into Dziekanski's death. One of them was Vincent Di Maio, an expert witness on tasers and a gunshot wound specialist. Di Maio also testified in the defence of George Zimmerman, who claimed that he shot seventeen-year-old Trayvon Martin in self-defence and was acquitted of second-degree murder and manslaughter in July 2013. The police officers who attended the scene at Vancouver International Airport also referred to excited delirium. Constable Rundel believed that Dziekanski had the condition: 'There's all these physiological characteristics that are going on within their body, and they're basically, for lack of a better word, they're on this downhill spiral towards expiring.' Constable Millington said, 'what I saw with regards to him being sweaty and his eyes really wide, and I think I said clammy in my notes as well, [...] that agitated state is very typical of someone who is – who has excited delirium'.

But in his inquiry Justice Braidwood cautioned against the use of a medical diagnosis that failed to explain how Dziekanski died:

> Ascribing a death to 'sudden death during restraint' gives no greater insight into the underlying medical cause of death than would 'sudden death during a car accident.' The same can be said for 'excited delirium.' It may be a convenient label to cluster frequently recurring physical conditions and activities, but offers no guidance as to the underlying physiological mechanisms that caused the death.

More than five years after the incident, Dziekanski's death was ruled a homicide by the British Columbia coroner's service.

Zofia Cisowski, Robert Dziekanski's mother, died in November 2019, during her annual visit to her home country. She was buried next to her only son. In 2010, she had created a memorial scholarship in his name at a local university in Kamloops, British Columbia, for geography students with Polish roots.

★

Charles Wetli might have played a crucial role in the evolution of
excited delirium in the medical establishment, but stakeholders
elsewhere have taken the diagnosis further than he ever could
have. Taser International, Inc. – renamed Axon Enterprise, Inc. in
2017 – had paid tens of thousands of dollars at a time to medical
examiners who testify on their behalf – Dr Charles Wetli was one
of them.

Since 2000, more than a thousand people in the US have died
shortly after being stunned with a taser – a gun-shaped device
which delivers a high-voltage, low-current electrical charge.
These devices fire electrified darts or barbs, causing pain and
neuromuscular paralysis – voluntary movement is disrupted and
the person is incapacitated. In 'drive stun' mode, the gun is held
directly against someone's body and then 'shot' to deliver a painful
shock, rather like a cattle prod.

A 2021 safety notice from Axon states that taser smart weapons
have been deployed over four million times, saving 257,195 lives
'from death or serious bodily injury' where more lethal measures
could have been used. The company's source for these figures is a
study that examined deaths that occurred in the context of stun-
gun use between 2001 and 2006. One of the authors of this study
was a paid member of Taser International's advisory board. The
company also states that in '1,201 field cases of taser use, 99.75%
resulted in no serious injury'.

Proponents of conducted energy devices (CEDs), of which
tasers are the most widely used, say that they are less likely to cause
injury and are less lethal than firearms, and that they minimise the
need to resort to firearms in the first place. Amnesty International
agrees with this basic premise but in practice, they say, CEDs are
rarely used as an alternative to firearms.

An extensive investigation by Reuters revealed that between

2000 and 2017, excited delirium has been listed as a factor in at least 176 deaths that followed taser use.

Axon holds hundreds of seminars for law enforcement each year. Their publications state that excited delirium makes people especially 'susceptible to the effects' of their devices. So does 'drug intoxication […] and/or over-exertion from physical struggle'.

In 2002, Taser provided the police with this statement, to be used when a fatality occurred following the deployment of a taser stun gun: 'We regret the unfortunate loss of life. There are many cases where excited delirium caused by various mental disorders or medical conditions, that may or may not include drug use, can lead to a fatal conclusion.' 'We're not telling departments [that] excited delirium is always the cause of death following a taser application,' said a spokesperson in 2007. 'We're simply pointing out the facts: that excited delirium is an issue out there, and they need to treat this as a medical emergency if they see these signs.'

Excited delirium is cited time and time again by US medical examiners, including in the cases of victims such as Keith Graff, who died in 2005, aged twenty-four, in Phoenix, Arizona, having been tasered for an uninterrupted 84 seconds; Roger Holyfield, who died in 2006, aged seventeen, in Jerseyville, Illinois (tasered twice as he carried a Bible, shouting 'I want Jesus'); Robert Knipstrom, who died in 2007, aged thirty-six, in Chilliwack, Canada (confronted with pepper spray, a metal baton and a taser); Efrain Carrion, who died in 2010, aged thirty-five, in Middletown, Connecticut ('shocked […] 34 times with a taser after he was handcuffed', according to a lawsuit); and Natasha McKenna, who died in 2015, in Fairfax County, Virginia, aged thirty-seven (wrestled by six deputies, handcuffed, placed in shackles and a spit hood, and tasered four times).

The relationship between Taser/Axon and US medical examiners is undeniably complex. In a 2011 survey, 13.5% of medical examiners admitted that they had changed a report in the past because of fear of litigation, even though only one in 221 respondents had actually been sued by the makers of the taser. A third of respondents said that the threat of litigation could affect their future decisions.

They may have been influenced by a 2006 case in which the company, then Taser International, sued the Ohio medical examiner Lisa Kohler. Kohler had ruled that taser shocks were contributory to the deaths of three men – Dennis Hyde, Richard Holcomb and Mark McCullaugh. Following a Summit County court order, references to stun guns were removed from the autopsy findings. For McCullaugh, 'homicide' was switched to 'undetermined', and a prison officer who was facing murder charges was acquitted. For Holcomb and Hyde, the cause of death was changed from 'homicide' to 'accidental'; in both cases, it was now found that they had entered 'crazed states consistent with excited delirium syndrome'.

The president of NAME described the Ohio case as 'dangerously close to intimidation […] we adamantly reject the fact that people can be sued for medical opinions that they make [*sic*]'. The company has repeatedly denied using intimidatory tactics, and state that they 'remain committed to our ongoing strategy of aggressively defending this type of litigation'. *

---

* Other critics have been sued for defamation and product disparagement, as reported by Reuters in their far-reaching investigation 'Shock Tactics: inside the taser, the weapon that transformed policing'. One example is the 2005 case of the Indiana medical examiner Roland Kohr, who stated that a taser played a contributory role in the death of James Borden. After being sued by Taser, he countersued and was issued with settlement terms: 'Dr. Kohr shall cease and desist from any negative comments, statements, publications, articles, manuscripts, interviews, or oral or written utterances of any type regarding Taser, its products, services, or personnel.' See Tim Reid and Paula Seligson, 'Taser's defense tactics include lawsuits against coroners and experts', Reuters, 24 Aug 2017.

The diagnosis of excited delirium is shepherded towards the police precinct as well as the pathology lab. Police1.com, a US site that claims 'more than 2 million visitors per month and over 650,000 registered members', offers '200 courses and 1,000 [...] training videos that are accredited or accepted for training in 37 states'. The site is 'used by more than 1,500 police departments', Police1.com reports, 'including the NYPD, Indianapolis Metro, and the entire state of Colorado'. It carries several articles on excited delirium. One describes it as a condition associated with a high percentage of arrest-related deaths, often requiring physical restraint and emergency sedation: 'Once the decision to do this has been made, action needs to be swift and efficient, and performed with all responders present when feasible.'

One of the authors of this piece is Jeffrey Ho, at the time medical director of Axon. Another is Mark Kroll, who was on Taser's Scientific and Medical Advisory board from 2003 and has testified as an expert for them in wrongful death suits, on one occasion stating: 'If you start exhibiting excited delirium behavior and you are in the terminal throes of death, and you are so bizarre you can't be controlled anyplace else, you will receive taser therapy [...]. They need to be brought under control so their lives can be saved.' Within six years of his appointment to Taser's board, *Mother Jones* reported in 2009, he had 'cashed in at least $2.5 million in company stock options', while Jeffrey Ho received '$70,000 during a recent 12-month stretch'. Reuters discovered that Kroll 'earned $267,000' from the company in 2016 alone. He remains an independent director of Axon, and according to the investment website Wallmine his share holdings were worth over $3 million as of August 2021.

Although the use of CEDs is especially common in the US, it increased by 37% in England and Wales in 2019–20 compared to the year before, although they were not discharged in 86% of these incidents (instead they were frequently drawn or aimed). The Home Office recently paid out for another 8,000 CEDs. In London alone, almost a third of Met police officers will carry CEDs by 2022. However, as we saw earlier in this chapter, when it comes to restraint the issue is not only how often CEDs are used but also against whom they are used. In 2020, the Home Office reported that

> CED use [again, referring to both discharge and non-
> discharge incidents] involved someone perceived as
> being from a Black ethnic group at a rate seven times
> higher than someone perceived as being from a White
> ethnic group in England and Wales (excluding the
> London Metropolitan police), and at a rate five times
> higher in the Metropolitan police force area.

It noted that, when combined with the rest of the national figures, the proportionately greater number of BAME people within the Metropolitan police force area compared to the rest of England and Wales 'can skew' the national picture. Whether diagnoses of excited delirium will rise in parallel with the increasing use of CEDs in the UK remains to be seen. But the emerging pattern from the US should serve as a warning.

The medical establishment may have conceived of excited delirium as a diagnosis, but it has been supported and endorsed by forces beyond it. And that is the reality of any diagnosis. It can at times explain, at times exonerate. The diagnostic process may start in the clinic, but it can end up in a courtroom. And it is to the courtroom that I'm going to travel next.

A 2006 US survey of a potential jury pool found that 46% expected to see some kind of scientific evidence in every criminal case. With excited delirium, that expectation can be met.

In 2009, Deborah Mash, Professor of Neurology and Molecular and Cellular Pharmacology at the University of Miami, authored a paper with colleagues which reported that there were distinct differences on post-mortem between people labelled with excited delirium and people who had died of other causes (such as cocaine intoxication or trauma).

Mash and her colleagues appeared to have uncovered something transformative: a pathological signature that could definitively identify someone who had died from excited delirium rather than excessive restraint. Excited delirium victims, the researchers found, had an increase in the expression of heat shock proteins. This was measurable at autopsy within twelve hours of death – get the body on a slab quickly, and the answers will lie within the gelatinous substance of the brain.

These victims also seemed to exhibit a decrease in dopamine transporters – another type of protein. This, Mash told the *New Scientist*, meant that victims who experienced a dopamine surge – if they were under stress or had taken drugs – were not able to clear the excess. 'Whether it's environmental stress or the crack pipe, it's going to trip the switch.' Such an overload of dopamine, she suggested, could cause cardiac malfunction and an inability to regulate one's body temperature, leading to sudden death.

The *Miami New Times* reported that in 2009, the same year as this research was published, Mash had earned $16,000 from Taser for her expert testimony. She told the newspaper that they had not funded her research, but refused to disclose her earnings from Taser before or since. Further court records showed Mash was paid around $24,000 for expert testimony in eight lawsuits filed in 2005–09. In these testimonies, she says she was trained by Charles Wetli. She calls him a 'mentor'.

In 2012, another group of researchers robustly disputed Mash's theory. Instead, they determined that these heat shock proteins were increased significantly in cocaine abusers, irrespective of the presence or absence of so-called excited delirium. But Mash's original findings had already been extrapolated from pathology lab to police station. In the case of one Florida teenager, those findings would shape how excited delirium featured in the story of his life and death.

In 2013, the skateboarder and graffiti artist Israel Hernandez-Llach had a fatal cardiac arrest after being shot with a taser stun gun. He was eighteen years old. Within four hours, Miami Beach Police Department received an email from Taser. That email, unearthed during the Reuters investigation published four years later, carried instructions on how to collect hair and nail samples from Hernandez-Llach's body, guidance on how to document his behaviour before he was tasered, and a sample press release for deaths involving taser devices. It also advised the Miami-Dade County Associate Medical Examiner to send Hernandez-Llach's brain tissue for testing to Deborah Mash.

In a section labelled 'Timely and Urgent', the email advises Daniel Morgalo, a Miami Beach police lieutenant who was himself a paid 'master instructor' for Taser, that his county medical examiner must be informed about the need to liaise with the 'cutting edge research centre' at the University of Miami Brain Endowment Bank, where 'Deborah Mash is the lead researcher on this matter'. The email provides Mash's contact details, emphasising, in an underlined sentence, that 'It's imperative to get this info to the ME [medical examiner] as the brain tissues must be collected ASAP.'

Mash determined that Llach's brain showed 'biomarkers consistent with excited delirium syndrome'. His death, according to her report, was consistent with the syndrome because of these biomarkers 'in conjunction with his elevated postmortem temperature, the physical exertion from running and the past use of psychotropic drugs and marijuana'. His toxicology was, in fact, negative for stimulants or hallucinogens, but Mash added that 'not every drug is detectable, particularly synthetic drugs'. She added that she was not providing an opinion on cause of death but rather furnishing 'an expert scientific opinion regarding the presence or absence of biomarkers and symptoms that are consistent with excited delirium syndrome'.

Although the Associate Medical Examiner determined that the cause of death was 'sudden cardiac death due to a conducted energy device discharge', the same examiner ruled the death as accidental. Nobody was charged.

22 August 2011.

The CCTV footage is grainy.

First, the camera from the police van shows 25-year-old Jacob Michael running away from his Cheshire home, chased by two police officers. Out through the white garden gate, up to the top of the road. Earlier, he had told his father that he had been threatened with a gun. He had called 999, but remained silent on the call before hanging up. Officers arrived at his home at 5.10 p.m., citing 'welfare concerns after an abandoned emergency call'. The atmosphere changed quickly, his father said later: 'They were so aggressive, saying, if you don't open the door, we're going to break it down. Very scary. Threatening.' The officers entered his bedroom and used pepper spray (they reported that they had been threatened with a hammer). Jacob said: 'Please don't, I'll do anything, please don't.' Then he ran. The next few minutes aren't captured on camera, but an inquest later hears that he is restrained by officers on the street. Batons were used. He calls for the police, because he does not believe that these people are the police. His hands are tied behind his back and his legs are strapped together.

The *Guardian* reports that 'Smith said one officer had his knee on Jacob's head, pushing his face into the road.'

Now Jacob re-emerges on CCTV. He is being loaded into the police van, wearing only white boxer shorts: his trousers have been pulled down to around his ankles during the fracas. He says 'sorry' at least four times. 'Please,' he says. 'Please.' His breathing is laboured.

Next clip: he is taken out of the van at the station. 'Stand up mate, we're not carrying you, stand up. On your feet.' But in the end, four officers carry him face-down into the building, each holding an arm or leg.

Holding Room 2. He is being held face to floor. One officer has placed a foot on Jacob's body. So has another. Six minutes go by. His body becomes still.

Then: frantic attempts by police officers and a nurse to resuscitate him.

Forty-five minutes after Jacob called for the police, he is pronounced dead. He is still handcuffed. His legs are still in restraints. INQUEST, an independent charity working with families bereaved by 'state-related' deaths, later issued a statement that opened with the words: 'Yet again, we begin an inquest into a death following restraint in police custody of a young black man.'

A Home Office pathologist reported that Jacob had died of excited delirium.

An inquest later heard that Jacob had taken cocaine during the weekend before his arrest and had been agitated after a weekend of partying. But his father was certain that Jacob never posed a threat to anybody else. He told the *Guardian*: 'He did nothing wrong, he hadn't committed any crime, he rang the police for help.' He and his wife had begged the officers to call an ambulance, and then 'my wife told them [...] that when they get to the police station to have a doctor to see him first thing. He looked so unwell, he was motionless, after they hit him with batons.' An inquest jury recorded a verdict of death by misadventure.

Kate Maynard is the solicitor who represented Jacob's family. She tells me that some of her cases, Jacob's included, have highlighted that delays in getting emergency medical care, prolonged restraint and the escalating use of force are all factors that ultimately contributed to these deaths.

Since the diagnosis of excited delirium risks characterising victims as hostile, crazed aggressors, how can law enforcement begin to identify someone like Jacob as needing urgent medical care rather than pepper spray, batons and handcuffs?

Dr Meng Aw-Yong, an A & E doctor and forensic medical examiner, tells me that using a term other than excited delirium might be the answer. The term he advocates is acute behavioural disturbance (ABD). He has co-authored the guidance on ABD for the Royal College of Emergency Medicine, and as the medical director for the Metropolitan Police Service in London he also plays an instrumental role in getting ABD into the vernacular of every police officer in the city.

ABD, says Aw-Yong, refers to a spectrum of behaviours, signs and symptoms, often presenting as a sudden onset of aggressive, bizarre, violent conduct and paranoia with profuse sweating, excessive strength, fast breathing, dilated pupils and 'inappropriate state of undress'. ABD, the guidelines state, usually occurs in the setting of acute or chronic drug or alcohol misuse and/or serious mental illness.

If this sounds to you rather like excited delirium, what with its superhuman strength and overheating and apparent violence and adrenaline surge – well, so it does to me. If it walks like excited delirium and talks like excited delirium, why should it be anything else? UK inquests have used ABD and excited delirium interchangeably.* But Aw-Yong argues that ABD should be seen as a call to action rather than a diagnostic label. He is keen to emphasise that ABD is not excited delirium:

> Excited delirium came from America because there
> was a huge explosion in the use of 'ice' – crystal
> methamphetamine. All these people started going crazy.
> American police tend to be more gung-ho, I think, in
> restraining people and so they were getting deaths. [The
> term] excited delirium was used for this behaviour.

Recognising the presence of ABD, he believes, could save lives. Police officers should identify ABD early, minimise restraint, which is especially dangerous in this situation, then call in medical help – ideally get paramedics on the scene, or take the patient to an emergency department rather than a custody suite. 'This is a medical emergency; it is not a policing emergency. People are dying.'†

---

* In 2020, the Forensic Science Regulator (FSR) issued guidance to pathologists in England, Wales and Northern Ireland on post-mortem reporting, advising pathologists to 'consider an approach where the central cause of the fatal clinical condition is offered as an immediate cause of death [e.g. amphetamine intoxication] and, where appropriate, used in conjunction with a term capturing the altered physiological and psychological state [e.g. ABD]'. […]. Discussions of excited delirium can still be included but 'may be better covered within the commentary section of the post-mortem report'. See 'Guidance: The Use of "Excited Delirium" as a Cause of Death', 231, Issue 2 (Birmingham: FSR and the Royal College of Pathologists, 2020), p. 5.

† Aw-Yong believes prompt medical attention could save these patients from a state called metabolic acidosis. 'If you over-exert yourself during a struggle or running around your adrenaline surges and you use up

Aw-Yong is not averse to the use of tasers (or other conducted energy devices), because he believes they minimise the need for physical restraint, which he sees as far more dangerous. He recognises that it's a controversial view: 'A lot of people are very scared of tasers, their misuse in some cases is terrible in the States, but it is reasonably well controlled here in the UK. If you use tasers to stop someone fighting, then the medics can get in and treat them earlier.'*

Kate Maynard agrees that using the term ABD and recognising it as a medical emergency could help to save lives and might have helped Jacob. 'The police training should, but by no means always does, ensure that all police officers have an ABD alarm bell for a medical emergency, and the need for de-escalation,' Maynard tells me. Her experience of coroners' cases has led her to believe that other services – ambulance, probation, emergency medicine staff – should train staff to recognise ABD, view it as a medical emergency and ensure an appropriate medical response.

Justifying a label – in this case, ABD – on the basis that it signals the need for urgent medical help is nothing new. In the key 2009 document on excited delirium from the ACEP, the task force

---

energy and oxygen,' he explains. 'The by-product of this is more carbon dioxide and hydrogen ions in your system, which through a series of reactions makes your body more acidic.' This state of metabolic acidosis has a whole host of consequences, including increased potassium in the blood, which catastrophically affects the heart rhythm, potentially causing death. Cocaine and some antipsychotic drugs can exacerbate heart strain. Restraint itself too can cause muscle breakdown, which ultimately can lead to kidney failure. The answer to all of this, he says, is to sedate these patients, reverse their metabolic acidosis, and correct the abnormal potassium levels in their blood.
* He has confirmed that he does not have any conflict of interest in relation to Axon. He is not paid by them, nor is he involved in delivering their training seminars.

(which included Jeffrey Ho and Deborah Mash) defined excited delirium as a 'true medical emergency' in its opening paragraphs. The word 'medical' appears close to forty times in the document. Excited delirium is described as a 'dangerous medical situation', a 'medical emergency' and a 'potentially medically unstable situation'. Law enforcement officers, the guidelines state, 'should recognize that ExDS subjects are persons with an acute, potentially life-threatening medical condition' and that emergency medical services should be called.

Aw-Yong's bid for change may be admirable, and it is supported even by the legal representatives of victims who have died under restraint. But over a decade ago excited delirium was also being framed as a medical emergency, one that needed medics as much as law enforcement. Look where that has got us.

Mikey Powell's cousin Tippa sighs in despair when I ask for his opinion on ABD: 'All of these things are used to detract, in my view, from the real issue, which is the method of restraint that was used.'

He believes there is another way to improve the fate of those confronted by police, without the use of yet another diagnostic label such as ABD. After Mikey's death, he moved to Birmingham to launch a campaign in his memory.

> I said to myself then that it's important to protest and people need to have the right to do that. But that cannot be the only tool in your bag. Standing outside stations and waving banners and shouting things is a good release for people, but sometimes the louder you shout, the more they don't hear. The only way to bring about change is to sit at the table and negotiate about how we try and improve things.

He worked with West Midlands Police, the local mental health trust, the ambulance service and several other organisations to develop a street triage programme, which began in 2014, for emergency call-outs involving someone who is believed to be experiencing a mental health issue. 'It's a team of specially trained police officers who have gone through mental health training. There's also a paramedic and a mental health or drug and alcohol officer, depending on the call. The vehicle has blues and twos, but it is unmarked or an ambulance.' The service ensures that vulnerable people with mental health needs are taken to a hospital setting if needed, rather than a police station.

In the first fourteen months of its operation, there was a 57% reduction in Section 136 detainments.* This sort of detainment, a form of arrest, does not require a warrant, and allows a police officer to bring a person who 'appears to be suffering from a mental disorder and is in need of immediate care or control' to a place of safety such as an emergency department. Only five people (of 2,356 incidents attended by the triage team) were taken into police custody following Section 136 use across the West Midlands Police area. The success of this programme seems to show us a way forward that does not rely on a diagnostic label. 'There have been no controversial restraint-related police custody deaths since triage launched in 2014,' says Tippa. '[Of] hands-on restraint cases like Mikey's, there hasn't been one. This program has saved lives.'

The influence of stakeholders outside the medical establishment can be transformative for a diagnosis, for better or worse. As we'll discover in the next chapter, another group of stakeholders

---

* Of nine subsequent similar pilot schemes across England, six sites showed a reduction in Section 136 detainments, with a mean reduction of 21.5% between them. See B. Reveruzzi and S. Pilling, *Street Triage* (London: UCL Press, 2016).

– patients and their families – is gathering to drive diagnoses forwards, to see their illnesses recognised, and symptoms treated.

Standing outside Thornhill police station, I remember the footage of Mikey Powell, motionless on the floor of the holding cell as *The Dogs of War* blared in the background. I remember the footage of Jacob Michael; 'Sorry' he says, repeatedly, minutes before his death. I remember Robert Dziekanski, convulsing on the airport floor when he had been on the brink of starting a new life in Vancouver. And now I remember George Floyd in his final moments: 'They're going to kill me', and 'Please, I can't breathe,' he gasped, and begged for his mother. 'My stomach hurts'; 'my neck hurts'; 'everything hurts'. Understanding the impact of a diagnosis often reveals who shapes it, and to what end. As Mikey Powell's family, and many other families like his, discovered, a diagnosis of excited delirium served everyone but him. These people, and their families, deserved so much better.

6

The Lost Children

'I can tell you exactly. It was March 22nd, 2016 at 5.45 in the evening and it was an absolute, abrupt decompensation,' says Georgia. 'So I contact the paediatrician and say, "Look, something has happened, my son has become feral, he'll only talk through my daughter, he keeps dropping to the floor."'

Georgia had already made the diagnosis herself, two years before, when her then twelve-year-old son Finn (not his real name), developed abnormal movements in his arms and legs within hours of an ear infection. 'I googled "acute onset involuntary movements" and PANDAS came up. I said to the doctor, "My son has got PANDAS, I know it's PANDAS, he needs antibiotics."'

PANDAS – paediatric autoimmune neuropsychiatric disorders associated with streptococcal infections – is a condition where children suddenly develop obsessive-compulsive disorder and/or tics. Within hours or days, their bodies begin to writhe, their limbs jerk, they fidget and stumble and sway into a new existence of perpetual motion. 'It was his shoulder, neck, his head, his trunk, his limbs, everything,' Georgia remembers. In PANDAS, even when symptoms seem to dissipate, they can return just as quickly. As the name suggests, the onset or exacerbation of symptoms are time-locked to a streptococcal infection. Georgia, a nurse, is unequivocal. She dated Finn's symptoms back to that ear infection, so she believed that this latest feral episode called for antibiotics.

A doctor agreed to give Finn an antibiotic – cefalexin – and she says that within four hours his symptoms had already started to improve. Five days later, 'there was a 90–95% reduction in symptoms [...].You know, the cefalexin brought him back.'

Despite Georgia's conviction, PANDAS is a condition that has engendered divisive debate. It is a contested diagnosis, the term for a condition for which there seems to be no medical explanation, or at least disagreement about whether the condition is medical or psychiatric. Some believe it is a 'real' disease, others do not. Either way, accusations swirl – of vested research interests, medical negligence, even child abuse.

Advocates of the diagnosis believe that children with PANDAS have a problem with their immune system which merits antibiotics, and sometimes heavy-duty immunomodulatory drugs, lifelong strict dietary restrictions and dialysis–type procedures. Families tell me they feel compelled to seek treatment on the fringes when the mainstream medical establishment rejects the diagnosis, even as they cling to information leaflets from PANDAS advocacy associations, even as they brandish newspaper stories of miracle recoveries: '"Exorcist" kids: the kids turned into strangers by bug mistaken for mental illness – that can be cured with antibiotics' ran a headline in *The Sun* in October 2018.

Finn was sent to a specialist and received a diagnosis of Tourette's, a condition of tics that is usually managed with talking therapy and primarily psychiatric drugs. Georgia disagreed, and eventually a friend of hers lent the family £10,000 which they used to take Finn to the US. 'This is classic PANS,' a doctor there told them (PANS, pediatric acute-onset neuropsychiatric syndrome, is a condition that is closely related to PANDAS but does not require proof of a streptococcal infection). She prescribed antibiotics and suggested that his symptoms might respond to a blood product called intravenous immunoglobulin – a treatment made from the pooled plasma of a thousand or more blood donors, usually used for blood cancers like leukaemia and myeloma, clotting disorders and critical immune deficiencies. Finn had been given the diagnosis that his mother had believed in all along.

Those who question the diagnosis of PANDAS, or believe it is wholly psychiatric, warn of the consequences of prolonged and aggressive treatment regimens. These children might, they argue, benefit at most from treatment for obsessive compulsive disorder – cognitive behaviour therapy, with or without psychiatric medications. In 2017, Georgia's son disclosed to a doctor in his mother's absence that she had taken him to the US for treatment. Georgia denies she withheld this information: 'At no point did I conceal anything, ever, to a professional. I would not.' A social worker was sent to the house, seemingly because fears had been expressed by the medical team that her son was the victim of fabricated or induced illness (FII), formerly known as Munchausen syndrome by proxy – a form of abuse where a child is presented for medical attention with symptoms and signs that have been fabricated or induced by their carer. This fear was never raised with her explicitly. She told the social worker: 'I will do it again, just so you know, I will get him out of this country. I will do it, so do your best, get your best evidence [for FII].' Georgia tells me that a safeguarding investigation concluded there were no concerns about her son's welfare. He has, to date, not received intravenous immunoglobulin.

Caught in a storm cloud of dispute, at some point in the future PANDAS will either stand or fall, will either lose validity or gain legitimacy. Families will either encounter acceptance of the diagnosis, and their children will receive antibiotics and immune treatments; or these families will continue to contend with scepticism and accusations, and their children will be directed instead towards psychiatrists, psychologists and social workers.

At the heart of it all, of course, are children who are unwell – regardless of the diagnostic label they receive. Finn is now eighteen. Cefalexin might have settled that feral episode, but he has had symptoms off and on ever since, Georgia explains. At one point, 'there was hostility and anger, and he kind of would lean to one side looking sideways, looking out of the corner of his eyes at us, as if we were doing something to him, as if we were harming him in some way'. She worries about the long-term impact. 'My son is a lot better than he was. A lot, lot better. But he still requires treatment. He's eighteen and he's incredibly clever, incredibly bright, he's had to give up [the subject he was studying] because of the interference of the OCD [obsessive-compulsive disorder]. So his life is a mess, he was three years out of school. He is quite depressed.'

In co-founding the PANS PANDAS UK charity – she is now its chair – Georgia is standing up for her belief that other children should not have to go through what Finn and her family did, to secure a diagnosis and treatment. 'I borrowed £10,000, I spent all of our credit cards, and had to sell the house because I'm not going to give up.'

Will PANDAS ever reach mainstream recognition? Through speaking to Georgia and other families who have fought similar battles, I want to explore what it might take for any diagnosis to become accepted, and whether PANDAS might find that acceptance. And if so, should it?

As I reflect on the fate of these children, I keep in mind some of Georgia's parting words – those she would want the whole medical establishment to hear: 'Doctors and nurses are just people and they are fallible. I would say "You're not more important than me, this is just your career, you are not more than me. You have to listen. This is real."'

★

Contesting a diagnosis is not to deny that these children have debilitating symptoms, or that their parents are profoundly distressed – speaking to families from the PANDAS community, there can be no doubt of this.

In discussions around PANDAS, it is tempting to ask whether it is 'real' or not. In some ways, this is code for 'is it made up?' or 'is it actually psychiatric?' – where 'psychiatric' is taken to mean a condition of the mind, which is perceived all too commonly, and devastatingly, as less valid than one of the body. It's an approach that, I believe, does grave injustice to young people like Finn. When patients fail to receive a diagnosis, or receive a contested diagnosis, they can feel that the broader medical establishment, and society itself, does not recognise their suffering, even rejects it. More practically, a contested diagnosis means a tougher fight for practical support such as access to disability benefits, compensation, rehabilitation or educational allowances (advocacy groups for PANDAS have called for students to be given extended time during exams, frequent breaks during lessons, and safe spaces).

When I began to speak to interviewees for this chapter, I was broadsided by a warning. Some sources felt I should not hint at the existence of any controversy around PANDAS. Some who advocate for the acceptance of PANDAS stipulated acceptance as a condition of speaking. They argued that some prominent classification systems include PANDAS within their bullet points. They sent me consensus papers on the subject. I wondered if this reflected a stance of sorts from some in the community, unspoken or informal: do not allow anybody writing about PANDAS to imply that there is any controversy, since every time people read about controversy, the diagnosis will be doubted.

Ethically, I cannot deny or suppress the contentious issues swirling around PANDAS (and PANS). Indeed, other members of the same community vociferously asked me to *highlight* these disputes, to show the clashes they encounter and the battles they fight each day to get treatment for their children.

It is true that there are consensus guidelines and peer-reviewed papers. But the consensus guidelines for treatment have been authored by the PANS/PANDAS Research Consortium. Advocates argue that all doctors should familiarise themselves with the guidelines, but not all doctors have faith in those guidelines, and some disagree with their existence in the first place. For every peer-reviewed paper written by high-profile clinicians and researchers supporting the presence of PANDAS, there are many others arguing against facets of the diagnosis. Even the WHO's recent inclusion of the condition in the ICD does not mean that it will be diagnosed and treated without a shred of doubt.

In 2017, the American Academy of Pediatrics published an article calling it a 'disorder fraught with controversy': 'While there is no controversy [about the fact] that the children have debilitating OCD, there has been controversy about the cause of the disorder and how to treat it.' A self-proclaimed 'believer' in the condition, Dr Michael Cooperstock, paediatric infectious diseases specialist at the Missouri School of Medicine, has acknowledged that 'as the field is emerging, the facts aren't all there, and so as long as the picture isn't scientifically completely filled in, there's room for disagreement.' Even the person who first coined the diagnosis – Susan Swedo of the US National Institute of Mental Health – has said that 'the main reason PANDAS/PANS is not diagnosed more is because of almost 20 years of controversy'.

And yet news reports do not always highlight these divisions or debates. On 25 January 2019, the BBC News site ran a story titled: 'Mother's Appeal After Boy Diagnosed with Autism When He Just Needed Antibiotics'. A few months before, on 24 September 2018, *The Times* had featured a story headlined 'Doctors miss child illness that alters personality'.

It is an emotive issue. When Donald Gilbert, a paediatric neurologist at the Cincinnati Children's Hospital in Ohio, gave a presentation to fellow medics which included the words 'Inoculate the family with education so they do not seek out a PANDAS/PANS clinic', complaints gathered beneath a video of the presentation that was posted on Facebook. The PANDAS network posted a call to action. In 2018, it advised that anyone who did not receive 'adequate care for your child or [if] you are concerned about his recent grand rounds presentation' should file complaints with the State Medical Board of Ohio, and that they should report a 'patient safety event' to the Joint Commission. Links to these forms were included with talking points and extensive instructions on how to complete them.

Replies to the post included:

'Done! Received my Complainant Decision to Pursue Dr. Gilbert letter today! If Dr. Gilbert won't answer to PANDAS parents, perhaps he will answer to the accreditation council!'

and

'YES! and don't be critical of how people chose [sic] to advocate – we all have one goal in mind. As they say there are many ways to skin a cat.'

I am not aware that any complaints made by the PANDAS community against Gilbert were ever upheld; but these impassioned responses show how sensitive a subject this is.

As reported by the journalist Brendan Borrell in 2020, some months later Gilbert, who was due to attend a conference, was warned by the event organisers to register at his hotel under a false name for his personal safety, and his name was left off the programme. Susan Swedo said she was offended that she had been 'compared [...] to a quack' in his presentation: 'I had grounds to sue him, but I chose not to.'

★

For any illness to be recognised in medicine, to be formalised and accepted, scientific evidence is part of the story. For contended and contentious diagnoses, miracle stories in newspapers are not enough. Scientific evidence can cement a diagnosis or decimate it. Find the supportive science, and a diagnosis thrives; if a theory is replete with logical fallacies, a diagnosis dies.

In the world of diagnosis, we favour an irrefutable mechanism to explain our diseases – the pathognomonic, i.e. characteristic, physical sign, the conclusive marker at autopsy, the definitive genetic abnormality *in utero* – these are the things that help to legitimise a diagnosis and secure its survival. Indisputable histological, biochemical and radiological signatures solidify an entity that is ephemeral – they give it ontological status and life and purpose. More than anything, we are convinced by the linkage of cause and consequence. It does not simply bring diseases and diagnoses to life; it makes them stick around. Conversely, contestable links make for contestable diagnoses, encircled by sceptics.

The PANDAS community places antecedent streptococcal infection at the core of the diagnosis. If that link were confirmed, its impact in securing the diagnosis would be enormous.

Take, for instance, the bacterium called *Vibrio cholerae*, which causes cholera. It plays an essential part in producing a disease – it must be present for the disease to occur, even though not all people carrying this bacterium will develop cholera. Likewise, the agent responsible for the infectious disease anthrax is *Bacillus anthracis*. If you have the symptoms of these infections and you test positive for these microorganisms, we can link your symptoms to the microorganism. This speaks to the concept of cause: an event or condition has preceded a disease event – without it, the disease would not have happened, or it would not have happened until sometime later. Epidemiologists also speak about 'necessary cause':

without a necessary cause, a disease does not occur – HIV is, by definition, a necessary cause of AIDS.*

Definitive links are not necessarily standard practice in medicine, though. Often, we must build support for a convincing case. We depend on finding associations and risk factors for diseases (like obesity for cancer) that are plausible and reproducible across multiple studies, with statistics that strongly support the argument, often with a documented temporal association between a preceding cause and effect, and a logic that fits with our existing scientific knowledge.

To locate this supportive science, many proponents of PANDAS have turned to another diagnosis that could support theirs, whose seemingly incontrovertible nature might pave the way to recognition.

Chorea Minor: Preliminary Report on Six Patients Treated with Combined ACTH and Cortisone.

Joseph Schwartzman, M.D., John B. Zaontz, M. D. and Henry Lubow, M. D., Department of Pediatrics, New York Medical College, Flower-Fifth Avenue Hospital and Metropolitan Hospital.

---

* There's another scientific concept drawn on by epidemiologists in the world of causality: sufficient-component cause. This is a minimum set of conditions or circumstances that, if present in a given individual, will inevitably produce the disease. No one component is sufficient on its own, but taken together they can provide a guarantee that an effect will occur. HIV infection can only occur following exposure to the HIV virus – it is a sufficient cause – but component factors also count, such as exposure to a person with HIV, unprotected sex, and the absence of HIV drugs that reduce the viral load of HIV.

Case 1. – M. S., a 7-year-old male, was admitted on
July 23, 1953 with a history that three weeks prior to
admission he began to manifest bizarre movements of
the right wrist and right lower extremity. He [...] began
to grimace, and his speech became slow and slurred.
Shortly thereafter the left upper and lower extremities
became involved. [...] Prior to this illness he had a
history of frequent respiratory infections including sore
throats. The family history revealed he had one sister
who had chorea and rheumatic carditis and his mother
had rheumatic heart disease. [...]
Case 2. – M. R., a 13-year-old Puerto Rican female,
was admitted on July 28, 1952, with a history of a
four-day illness with bizarre purposeless movements
of all extremities and difficulty in talking, with the
speech being muffled and slurred. [...] Upon physical
examination she manifested facial grimaces, snakelike
movements of the tongue, marked athetoid [writhing]
movements, muscular weakness, restlessness, and
irritability. [...] She also had a harsh blowing systolic
[cardiac] murmur over the mitral region.

Acute rheumatic fever usually occurs within weeks of a streptococcal sore throat and manifests with arthritis, cardiac inflammation
(and sometimes, later, rheumatic heart disease), a pink or red
rash and nodules under the skin. Up to a fifth of children with
rheumatic fever also develop abrupt random jerks in the arms
and legs, facial grimacing and twitches, a darting tongue, muscle
weakness, emotional outbursts, restlessness, and occasionally
features of obsessive-compulsive disorder. The condition, known
as Sydenham's chorea – or chorea minor, in earlier papers ('chorea'

derives from the Ancient Greek *choreia*, 'dance') — is thought to relate to a misdirected immune response. These children's immune systems produce antibodies — Y-shaped proteins — directed against the bacteria invading their systems. The antibodies then seem to cross-react with the antigens of their own nervous systems, because our antigens share structural similarities with the infectious agent — and so the overenthusiastic antibodies of the immune system can damage both the infectious agent and the body's nervous system. In Sydenham's chorea, the brain's movement centre — the basal ganglia — seems to bear the brunt of this assault, triggering off jerks and tics and twitches and grimaces. With penicillin treatment, children with Sydenham's chorea usually improve within three to four months, and most recover fully, although recurrences can occur.

The children with chorea in the aftermath of streptococcal infection described by Schwartzman and his colleagues were among many reported in the 1950s and 1960s, although hints at an association between 'rheumatism' and chorea had begun to form even in the early nineteenth century. In the early twentieth century, scientists injected bacteria taken from the cerebrospinal fluid of patients who had died with acute rheumatic fever into the brains of rabbits. Those rabbits developed irregular movements, cardiac disease and arthritis. Since then, the widespread and routine use of antibiotics for streptococcal infections, alongside improvements in living conditions, has decreased the incidence of Sydenham's chorea, at least in well-resourced settings.*

If a streptococcal infection is so convincingly linked to

---

* Acute rheumatic fever is still a major public health issue in low- and middle-income countries. Globally, there are half a million new cases of acute rheumatic fever each year and 275,000 deaths due to rheumatic heart disease alone.

Sydenham's chorea, why can't the same smooth line be drawn to PANDAS? Couldn't some children develop obsessive-compulsive symptoms or tics after an infection? That's one argument among advocates of the latter condition, but it's a contentious one: even in Sydenham's chorea, a definitive autoimmune process or antibody has never been established.

The story of PANDAS began in the 1980s, at the US National Institute of Mental Health in Bethesda, Maryland. Susan Swedo and her team, like investigators before them, had begun to identify frequent obsessive-compulsive features in children with documented rheumatic fever and proof of a positive time-locked streptococcal infection. In the 1990s, the group decided to change tack.

They started to examine children with obsessive-compulsive symptoms and tics, and looked backwards for a preceding strepto-coccal infection. That definition of a past infection was fairly tangential. Even an account of a sore throat counted – without any diagnostic test for a streptococcal infection – as did a past history of streptococcal throat or simple exposure to streptococcal infection through a past school outbreak. The researchers named this condition PANDAS, characterised by abrupt onset of OCD and/or tics. It made its official appearance in the *American Journal of Psychiatry* in February 1998. But assuming a definitive link between psychiatric symptoms and streptococcal throat is fraught with complications, as Swedo herself acknowledged. There are high background rates of strep throat infections in the community at a given time, and lots of children are carriers (around one in twenty) without any symptoms. Even if children do have streptococcal antibodies, that could simply suggest exposure to an infection from many months before – those antibodies tell us little about whether that infection is related to current symptoms or when that infection occurred, since antibodies remain elevated for more than a year in more than half of children. Added to that, cases of OCD are common at a given time (up to 4% of children), as are cases of tic disorders (up to 20% of children). So there is a reasonable chance that a child will have OCD *and* a past or current streptococcal infection simply because both things are common, not because one is caused by the other. The link is coincidental rather than causal.

A number of studies, including one that followed up children diagnosed with PANDAS for two years, failed to find evidence of a temporal association between streptococcal infections and an exacerbation of tics or obsessive-compulsive symptoms, or antibodies that might suggest an autoimmune process.

Failure to establish cause and consequence, or even a clear association, may sound the death knell for any diagnosis. If PANDAS turns out to have drawn an erroneous link between an infection and the clinical features of tics and compulsion, the vehemence of its dismissal could parallel the fervour of those who insist on its legitimacy and demand its acceptance.

What then, might be the way forwards? In recent years, the diagnostic criteria for PANDAS have been widened, with the introduction of the related syndrome PANS. These children abruptly and dramatically develop OCD or severely restricted food intake. There are other supportive features, such as irritability, aggression, severe oppositional behaviours and deterioration in school performance. A key difference between PANS and PANDAS is that PANS does not require those who diagnose it to find proof of a causative streptococcal infection. Instead, PANS occurs with no specified precipitant. It could happen, say those who have settled on this diagnostic label, in the context of another infection (perhaps Lyme disease, glandular fever or herpes), drugs, or as yet undefined environmental and metabolic triggers.* Worldwide PANDAS organisations have now been rebranded as PANS/PANDAS organisations.

A focus on PANS could circumvent the cause-and-consequence argument around streptococcal infections, and it has drawn a larger number of influential clinicians and researchers to these discussions. But equally, the lack of specificity is ripe for critique. Most importantly, a clinical picture that is so broad in scope could risk sending affected children down a rabbit hole of invasive investigations and treatments.

In the absence of a widely accepted line that can be drawn between cause and consequence, PANS and PANDAS advocates will need to secure their diagnosis through other means. Beyond antibodies and antigens, beyond cause and consequence. They must capture the attention of those at the highest level in the medical and political establishments.

In 2001, an American woman called Mary Leitao was trying to find a remedy for her son Drew, who was just under three years

---

* This was influenced by a large Danish study that examined the medical records of more than one million children. It found that the risk of developing mental disorders in children was increased by more than 80% after a hospitalisation for severe infection (the risk of OCD was eightfold in teenagers). The use of antibiotics to treat those infections was linked to a 40% greater risk of mental disorders. This is not proof that antibiotics themselves or, for that matter, the infections themselves cause mental disorders. Perhaps mental disorders were simply more likely to be identified in these children because they had ongoing interactions with doctors who asked about their well-being. Maybe infections and medication use were a proxy for social deprivation, which itself is linked to mental health disorders. Perhaps some of these children carried a genetic risk of infection which overlapped with a genetic risk of mental disorders.

old at the time and had an irritated patch of skin below his lip. He pointed to the patch now and then. 'Bugs,' he would say. His mother had tried eczema creams and scabies ointments, in vain. One evening, she later told the *Pittsburgh Post-Gazette*, she rubbed the latest cream into his skin only to see 'something fibre-like' emerge. Mary, a biologist, bought an $8 toy microscope the next day, examined the strange substance, and saw a solitary filament. More of these filaments – blue and red and black – emerged from Drew's skin over the following weeks and months.

With that toy microscope and with the discoveries she made, Mary scaled unimaginable heights. Her crusade to raise the prominence of the disorder she identified in her son could illustrate how PANDAS might secure the same coverage.

After discovering those fibres emerging from her son's skin, Mary went online and found kindred spirits there. These fibre-afflicted sufferers bathed in bleach and ingested deworming drugs at doses meant for cattle, to rid themselves of these bodily invaders. They picked at their skin, leaving disfiguring scars, they tweezed the fibres from their pores, they extracted them from follicles using nail-clippers. They had been dismissed by dermatologists, allergy doctors and infectious disease physicians. Some had been disowned by their own families. All they had was one another, online.

Mary named the condition 'Morgellons' after a description in a seventeenth-century letter by the physician and author Thomas Browne of 'that endemial Distemper of little Children in Languedock [*sic*], called the Morgellons, wherein they critically break out with harsh Hairs on their Backs, which takes off the unquiet symptoms of the Disease, and delivers them from Coughs and Convulsions'.

Sufferers of Morgellons disease report a constant crawling under their skin, feelings of itching, stinging, biting. Black sweat runs from their pores. Fibre-like structures — cactus-like, sometimes — sprout from their limbs and their faces. Occasionally, granules and black specks swim or scuttle beneath the skin, or hatch from it. Some patients claim that these are created by parasites, others regard them as foreign substances that cannot be classified. There are other symptoms too — fatigue and joint swelling, difficulty with concentration, and short-term memory loss.

Mary launched a Morgellons website and later the non-profit Morgellons Research Foundation (with herself as executive director), created a medical advisory board, and found sympathetic doctors and nurses – some of whom had the condition themselves. Soon, Morgellons extended its tentacles even deeper into her home life: her two other children developed symptoms in the aftermath of their father's sudden death.

Blog posts on the Morgellons Research Foundation site are a compendium of patients' distress and desperation. Some disclose their terror of infecting others: 'I can no longer hug a friend or kiss a lover. When my dog showed signs of this disease I had to let him go.' Others share stories of the devastating impact on their families: 'Last year, my eldest son bypassed his first-choice college and a $40,000 scholarship in favor of helping us by living at home.'

Psychiatrists agree these patients are distressed, but dispute theories of invading microbes. Instead, they call the condition 'delusional parasitosis' or 'delusions of parasitosis' (DOP) – a well-established type of psychosis that was named long before Morgellons. Psychiatrists explain that these filaments are simply fibres from patients' clothing; the welts and wounds arise through the scratching of an infernal itch. In the 1930s, textbooks included the 'matchbox sign' (and, later, the 'Ziploc sign') as a typical presenting feature of DOP: patients carry physical evidence cautiously into their medical appointments, as proof that they are not mad. These matchboxes, in the eyes of some medics, prove that they are. At conferences, many with Morgellons wear T-shirts with the letters 'DOP' scored out with a red line.

Dermatologists report that biopsies of these patients show normal skin, or simply an inflammation where people have scratched themselves. Sociologists characterise Morgellons as a mass delusion or mass psychogenic illness, facilitated online: 'The world wide web has become the incubator for mass delusion and [Morgellons] seems to be a socially transmitted disease over the internet.'

Mary continued to bring Drew to a series of doctors. One letter from a Johns Hopkins paediatrician concluded: 'Ms. Leitao would benefit from a psychiatric evaluation and support, whether Andrew has Morgellons disease or not. I hope she will cease to use her son in further exploring this problem.' Another physician raised the possibility of Munchausen's syndrome by proxy. There are echoes of the accusations lobbied at parents within the PANDAS community.

Delusional parasitosis was briefly alluded to in my training, but most of my exposure to the condition of Morgellons came later, from a dizzying array of newspaper features and TV documentaries in the last decade. The mobilisation of the Morgellons Research Foundation has taken on epic proportions, disseminating descriptions of this condition to the broader public and launching stories of true suffering to national and international media.

The diagnosis even haunted folk singer Joni Mitchell. In 2010, she described it to the *Los Angeles Times* as a 'weird incurable disease that seems like it's from outer space':

> Fibres in a variety of colours protrude out of my skin
> like mushrooms after a rainstorm: they cannot be
> forensically identified as animal, vegetable or mineral.
> Morgellons is a slow, unpredictable killer – a terrorist

disease: it will blow up one of your organs, leaving you
in bed for a year.

The Morgellons Research Foundation reached the next level
with a mailing campaign that mobilised top-ranking politicians,
as outlined by the journalist Will Storr in his 2011 article for
the *Guardian*, 'Morgellons: A hidden epidemic or mass hysteria?':
'Thousands have written to Congress demanding action. In
response, more than 40 senators, including Hillary Clinton, John
McCain and a pre-presidential Barack Obama, pressured [the
CDC] to investigate; in 2006, it formed a special taskforce, setting
aside $1m to study the condition.'

In 2007, the CDC removed delusional parasitosis from its
website, created a page titled 'Unexplained Dermopathy: "AKA
Morgellons"' and began to research the condition in earnest.

Morgellons, at least as it was conceived by Mary Leitao, had not
existed before 2002. At the last count, the Morgellons Research
Foundation had more than 14,700 families worldwide registered
in their database.

Patient power is influential. Movements like this one can secure
medical coverage, compensation and accountability. They can
shape public policy. They can afford a condition legitimisation.
Patient-led campaigns pushed for recognition of the links
between asbestos and lung cancer, and between birth defects
and thalidomide. Veterans of the Vietnam War, alongside some
sympathetic psychiatrists, pushed for the inclusion of PTSD in
psychiatric classification systems. There were other supportive
factors – emerging science, media backing and renegade clinicians
willing to speak out – but patients were instrumental in this
challenge to medical omnipotence and orthodoxy.

The CDC finally issued its findings in 2012. They did not meet
the Morgellons community's hopes. Researchers had examined

skin biopsies from 115 patients in northern California: there was occasional evidence of insect and spider bites, and sometimes chronic skin-picking and rubbing. Most fibres collected from participants' skin were composed of cellulose 'likely of cotton origin', or represented fragments of skin. Morgellons, the CDC concluded, shared a number of features with 'delusional infestation'.

Although the Morgellons campaigners reached the highest echelons of the medical and political establishments, the outcome of their efforts might still sound a warning bell for the PANS/PANDAS community. Ultimately, the Morgellons community was not granted the acceptance it had sought, and the condition remains firmly embedded in medical literature as delusional parasitosis.

In the UK, the PANS/PANDAS charity has embarked on similar activities to those of the Morgellons campaigners. They have established a physicians' network – drawing a number from prominent and reputable research institutes – organised conferences and created information leaflets for parents to take to their GPs and schools. They aim to meet with an all-party parliamentary group soon, Georgia tells me, and she points to an upcoming treatment trial for children with the diagnosis. But securing this level of interest might also secure heightened scrutiny and ultimately yield answers they do not wish to hear. Large-scale investigations from respected research bodies can challenge the legitimacy of a condition or simply deny it. At the very least, it might be deemed to be psychiatric rather than medical, which, in the eyes of Morgellons sufferers, invalidates their experiences.

Most families I speak to about their child's PANS or PANDAS believe that even if there are psychiatric symptoms, a medical cause underlies them – something neurological, something immunological, something 'real', one parent says, hopefully.

When her young daughter mentioned 'Finn's Tourette's' during one of his early episodes, Georgia turned to her and said: 'He hasn't got Tourette's, it's the immune system, it's neurological problems producing psychiatric symptoms. You must hold on to that. If anything happens to me, you must hold on to that, don't let them tell you otherwise.'

For Catherine, the mother of eleven-year-old Lucas, these concerns run similarly deep. She feels that a psychiatric diagnosis denies her truth and will deprive her son of a cure.

When I first speak to Lucas via a Zoom call in September 2020 (it's several months into the coronavirus pandemic and the family have only just emerged from shielding), he tells me about his return to school. 'Some of the stuff is different, we're not really doing clubs. There are loads of signs, and you have to wear a mask, not like the whole time, but there's one lesson for fifty minutes where you have to wear it because we're too close.'

He sits upright in a crisp, perfectly unruffled white shirt, confident and talkative. He tells me about the sports he plays, kindly and patiently explaining the more complex aspects of rugby and cricket (he plays for two local teams), and telling me of his dream to play rugby professionally for the Saracens.

There is little sign of any shadow cast by the events of April 2019. His mother Catherine has asked that I do not use the family's real names or specify the tropical island they had gone to on holiday, where it all began.

'I feel really weird, Mummy,' he said one morning on that holiday. She recalls that 'he threw himself onto the bed. I thought he was just hot, or he had had a bad night's sleep'. After a boating activity later that day, he went back to bed. 'When he woke up, he was just not our son. He was agitated, he was confused, he was angry, he was rude to the tour guide. He's normally never rude.' The family headed back to the mainland to find a doctor; during the trip,

Lucas became difficult to rouse. His father, Alex, carried him off the boat to a waiting ambulance. There, Lucas became agitated, was restrained by paramedics, and by the time he reached the hospital the situation had nosedived. 'It was like he was gone into an autistic, non-verbal bubble,' remembers Catherine. 'He couldn't see you. But then he would just start laughing, he was completely manic, and he'd scream. He was constantly tapping his fingers, whistling, singing songs over and over again. He was really obsessive about food, almost eating like an animal. He was being like a baby.'

He had some mosquito bites but no fever, and his blood tests did not show evidence of malaria or sepsis. A lumbar puncture and MRI did not yield any answers. Steroids, antivirals and antibiotics made no difference. At one point, Alex recalls, the medical team seemed to have only one option left. 'The doctor, who trained in the US and in a UK hospital, was excellent. He came in, he got the rest of the staff to come in, and said, "Would you mind if we do something? Do you mind if we pray for him?"'

Eventually, the team trialled an epilepsy drug – they had noticed that Lucas was staring blankly ahead at times. Over the next few days he began to improve, perhaps because of this treatment, perhaps not. By the end of the week, Lucas was himself again.

The improvement was short-lived. Within days of their return to England, the symptoms recurred – the finger-tapping and whistling and maniacal laughing – and his parents rushed him to A & E. 'Then he just started to sleep, to the point I thought we were losing him.' Catherine tells me that the doctors were ready to dispatch Lucas to a psychiatric ward, but she believes the family's intervention – they showed the consultant an email from an encephalitis specialist they had contacted, who said Lucas urgently needed neurological investigations – averted this outcome. Lucas was transferred to a tertiary hospital. He was initially treated with steroids, antivirals and antibiotics to cover the possibility of an autoimmune disorder, but Catherine tells me that on day seven they settled on a diagnosis of 'stress reaction to being sick on holiday'.

During the next few months after he was discharged, Lucas repeatedly experienced further episodes. Catherine describes how they 'would lose him for seven to nine days at a time. He was in an autistic bubble, he was drooling, his balance was off, he was holding his head to the side, he was completely cognitively altered, couldn't function, could not do anything for himself, he was just not there.' Since then, although there have been intervals of normality, there have also been 'frenzied' episodes of screaming, intermixed with trance-like states, and what Catherine thinks are hallucinations ('the other day he was stroking a blanket thinking it was a dog') and intrusive thoughts. Doctors have recommended psychological and psychiatric treatments – therapy and benzodiazepines. And yet, a psychiatric diagnosis simply has never made sense to the family, said Catherine.

At one point, they remembered a suggestion from a friend during Lucas's second UK hospital admission. 'My friend phoned me, and she said, "I think it is this condition, I've looked it up, what you're telling me."' That condition was called PANDAS. The family sought an opinion in the private sector. The doctor they saw agreed with the diagnosis – more specifically, the related condition of PANS, albeit an atypical version, they acknowledged, given 'the absence of OCD or restricted eating patterns'. More recently, an immunologist has dialled this down to 'an immune dysregulatory disorder – the results rule out a significant autoimmune disorder', but Lucas has still received antivirals, antibiotics and anti-inflammatories. At times they have helped, Catherine believes. Other times, it seems, less so. 'Recently, I introduced acyclovir [an antiviral] and within three days he's back to school, he's doing a lot better.'

I ask her why she is against PANS being classified as a psychiatric condition. 'I think it's very dangerous to give [a psychiatric] diagnosis, because it might stop those children being treated [with medications other than psychiatric drugs].' She also brings up the ineffectiveness of psychiatric medications. 'If PANS was a psychiatric diagnosis, then psychiatric medication could help it,' she says. 'We have been down the whole treatment with psych meds, they don't work, they make symptoms worse.'

A failure to respond to psychiatric treatment does not mean that a condition is not psychiatric, though: not everyone responds to psychiatric treatment for depression, but that does not necessarily mean it is not psychiatric. There is a wider discussion to be had here, about why we should distinguish between neurological and psychiatric disorders, between brain and mind, in the first place.

But it seems to me that, for parents, the acceptance of a diagnosis is not always, or at least not only, about the specific diagnosis itself, but about doctors acknowledging that their child is ill and suffering. 'I'm not [going] to doctors saying "please give me this diagnosis",' says Catherine. 'I'm past that point.' This sense of rejection manifests itself in the doubt and distrust they express at times: 'I'm just looking, constantly looking and double-checking if there's something they've missed,' Catherine says of some of the doctors Lucas has seen. Georgia also remembers scrutinising one neurologist who saw Finn: 'The history-taking was poor, in my experience, and it took her four minutes to do a neurological examination. I timed her, because at this point I had become vigilant, I am looking for their omissions.'

Both Catherine and Georgia allege that certain doctors they have met have vested interests that compromise their diagnostic abilities. Catherine says that one psychiatrist Lucas saw is involved in research that is out to challenge PANS: 'Her training is in OCD

190 The Imaginary Patient

and Tourette's, and if this whole thing [PANS] challenges her work, then it's difficult, she's so entrenched.'

Georgia echoes this sentiment with regard to bias within the medical community: 'If you go and see a neuro or paediatrician and they have a particular research interest, what you tell them conflicts with everything they know and understand and believe.'

I ask Lucas about his medications. 'I take them because I have to.' Does he know how many tablets? 'There's, like, three, or maybe … I don't remember how many.' Do they help? 'Yeah, maybe. I don't really realise.'

There are still many days when he hallucinates, Catherine says, and there have been days filled with frenzied screaming states and trances, when they simply cannot reach him. Today, thankfully, is not one of those days.

Beyond Lucas – although he knows little of it – there is a community fighting for the treatment it believes could change the lives of children like him, could heal the relentless tics and obsessions, terminate the endless compulsions and ferocious rages. The driving force is a hunger for treatment beyond what these parents believe psychiatry can offer. 'These children are trying to throw themselves out of windows and moving cars,' says Georgia. '[Psychiatrists] say CBT [cognitive behavioural therapy] is the panacea, it's the cure–all, an antipsychotic will resolve these symptoms, and they don't.' She has worked as a nurse in mental health herself. 'I've seen it myself in psychiatry; when the drugs no longer work, they don't work, and patients get worse. I saw very few people improve with psychiatric medication [once the medication stopped working].'

This desperation for a 'non–psychiatric' cure might capture the attention of another group, which, as clinical trials for PANDAS/ PANS begin, is ready to intercede.

★

Once upon a time, the pharmaceutical industry gave oxygen to a then disputed and marginalised diagnosis. Over the preceding years, before the industry stepped in, the disorder had inspired academic articles such as 'Pain is real; fibromyalgia isn't' from the editor of the *Journal of Rheumatology*, and '"Fibromyalgia" and the medicalization of misery'. Could the pharmaceutical industry, by adopting and championing PANS and PANDAS as it did fibromyalgia, similarly drive their acceptance in medical circles?

The rheumatologists Frederick Wolfe and Brian Walitt have traced the evolution of fibromyalgia over the last century or so, from neurasthenia – a condition of 'nervous exhaustion' and body pain first described in the nineteenth century, with which it shares certain features – to the similar syndrome of fibrositis known during much of the twentieth century (fatigue, pain, stiffness and soreness), and finally to the more refined definition of fibromyalgia in the 1980s and after. In 1990, formal classification criteria were developed by the American College of Rheumatology (ACR) – Wolfe was lead author on this paper – and included widespread pain as described by the patient, and specific points of tenderness as confirmed by a physician's examination. Detractors voiced concerns: 'Fibromyalgia has become a proposition so broad that it includes all possibilities,' wrote one rheumatologist. Yet the suffering of people diagnosed with fibromyalgia was not in question. In one study, patients with various chronic diseases were asked to complete a health-related 'quality of life scale'. People with fibromyalgia scored lower than people with chronic lung disease, rheumatoid arthritis or advanced cancer. The doubters who doubted the diagnosis could not doubt the illness.

In a remarkable about-turn, Frederick Wolfe told *The New York Times* in 2008 that he had become cynical and discouraged with regard to fibromyalgia, despite leading the ACR team that developed those key criteria: 'Some of us in those days thought that we had actually identified a disease, which this clearly is not. To make people ill, to give them an illness, was the wrong thing.' He and Walitt now believe that it is a psychocultural disorder, driven 'primarily by psychological factors and societal influences [...] there is as yet no compelling evidence that an underlying central nervous system disturbance contributes in a substantial or clinically meaningful way'.

Despite Wolfe's having stepped back from the diagnosis so dramatically, the train had already left the station. As he acknowledges, the status of fibromyalgia has been 'buttressed by social forces that include support from official criteria, patient and professional organizations, pharmaceutical companies, disability access, and the legal and academic communities'.

More than anyone on that list, it's the pharmaceutical industry which has led fibromyalgia's march towards acceptance by the mainstream. Its appetite is unsurprising, given that chronic widespread pain (that is, pain lasting at least three months) is present in about 10–15% of the population, of whom many will receive prescription drugs for their pain. The prevalence of fibromyalgia is thought to range between 2–6%, rising with age, and it is more common in women (the fervent rejection of the diagnosis by some might represent a pejorative view of female pain and distress, as much as an argument against the scientific credibility of the diagnosis).

In 2007, a medication called Lyrica, developed by Pfizer, was approved by the FDA (US Food and Drug Administration) for treatment of the syndrome. Lyrica is the trade name for a drug called pregabalin, which was already being used for epilepsy and neuropathic pain (nerve pain associated with diabetes and shingles); but a 2007 report estimated that the arrival of drugs specifically licensed for fibromyalgia would contribute to a quadrupling in size of this new drug market.

Pfizer teamed up with the US National Fibromyalgia Association (NFA) on an awareness campaign: an interactive website, a dedicated phone line for information on recommended drugs, and a public service announcement that strove to validate patients' experiences.

Endorsement of patients' suffering was a key component of the campaign. Lynne Matallana, the president of the NFA, told *The New York Times*: 'The day that the FDA approved a drug and we had a public service announcement, my pain became real to people.'

The sociologist Kristin Barker from Oregon State University dug into these advertising campaigns, and also scoured through patient forums, finding that patients there were relieved too. Of the Lyrica adverts, one said: 'It somehow validates us as human beings that have a debilitating illness not just the hypochondriacs they thought we were.' Advertisements from 2007 and 2008 emphasised that Lyrica was not an antidepressant – as if to refute any accusation that the disorder was 'all in the mind' – and encouraged viewers to 'ask your doctor about Lyrica today'. Nonetheless, some members of the fibromyalgia community were ultimately disillusioned by the ads, Barker discovered, concerned that if the drug failed to provide a miraculous response they would be regarded as fraudulent or hysterical, even by their own families.

Pfizer also prominently bolstered fibromyalgia research. A handful of publications existed on the disorder in 1980. By 2010, there were around 400 a year.

In 2007, Lyrica brought in $1.8 billion in revenue, an increase of 58% compared to 2006, the year before it was approved for fibromyalgia. By 2009, sales of the drug had reached $2.8 billion, and only sales of Lipitor – a statin drug used to treat high cholesterol – surpassed it in Pfizer's portfolio. Lyrica even outperformed Viagra.

Later, other medications were licensed for fibromyalgia, and in 2010 the market exploded when the diagnostic criteria for fibromyalgia were changed, so that they could be defined by patients' self-reported experiences alone – easily measured by a self-assessment questionnaire they would fill out in the waiting room, which confirmed their experiences of widespread pain, fatigue, unrefreshed sleep and cognitive difficulties ('fibro fog'), as well as somatic symptoms such as abdominal pain and cramps.

Direct-to-consumer advertising of prescription pharmaceuticals is not permitted in Europe (it is only legal in the US and New Zealand) but company-sponsored research papers were published internationally and disseminated in internet forums that spread the message far and wide. Selling drugs sometimes means selling diagnoses, across international borders too. In England and Wales, there was an eleven-fold increase in prescriptions for pregabalin between 2006 and 2016 (from 476,102 prescriptions to 5,547,560).

Although is not specifically licensed for fibromyalgia in the UK, the official NHS patient website advises that 'research has shown' that pregabalin 'can improve the pain associated with fibromyalgia in some people' and advises: 'If you think you have fibromyalgia, visit your GP.' This seems a little more optimistic than formal findings by the independent Cochrane network's review of eight studies that examined pregabalin:

> Pregabalin at daily doses of 300 to 600 mg produces a large fall in pain in about 1 in 10 people with moderate or severe pain from fibromyalgia [these results were similar to other medications for fibromyalgia, including milnacipran and duloxetine]. Pregabalin offers good pain relief to only a minority of people with fibromyalgia; it will not work for most people.

These drugs are not without risk. In her analysis, Barker found that advertisements for Lyrica were keen to direct the viewer's attention elsewhere: 'At the exact second that "suicidal thoughts and tendencies" are listed as a possible side effect, the screen fills with a burst of glorious sunshine coming through the trees engulfing the professor in a warm glow.'

Pregabalin was reclassified as a controlled substance in the UK in 2019, because of the risk of abuse and dependence. It carries potentially fatal interactions with alcohol and opioids. Pregabalin is increasingly implicated in poisoning deaths related to drug misuse. Between 2019 and 2020, there was as a 41% rise in fatalities (from 244 to 344 deaths) in England and Wales.

Barker draws on the idea of 'pharmaceutical determinism' in her work, that is, how the 'mere existence of a prescription medication for a condition is used to authenticate the biomedical existence and character of the condition itself'.

Fibromyalgia sceptics still exist, and patients are devastated to find a legacy of disbelief that lingers in the minds of healthcare professionals and lay people alike. One website carried a letter entitled: 'To the person who thinks my fibromyalgia isn't real'. There are legions of sufferers reporting a prolonged journey to receiving the diagnosis.

I wrote earlier about how the question of whether a diagnosis is 'real' or not does a disservice to those who are suffering: binary 'real–not real' judgements concerning the authenticity of a diagnosis invalidate the experiences of those who come forward with their accounts of distress. I'm struck by the ways in which a diagnosis is shaped and how those experiences of suffering are validated: it is largely because of intervention from the pharmaceutical industry (even though Pfizer has now lost its patent protection, and pregabalin generics have just been approved) that patients with widespread pain and fatigue have an increased chance of receiving a diagnostic label of fibromyalgia and medication such as pregabalin from their doctors. Not all doctors who prescribe pregabalin are fully on board with the existence of a biological substrate for the diagnosis, but even they are at least willing to compromise – by documenting the label and dispensing the medication. The 'Pain Is Real; Fibromyalgia Isn't'-editorials have disappeared, and when celebrities like Lady Gaga announce a diagnosis of fibromyalgia, they are broadly met with support rather than derision. Their illness, their suffering, is recognised – certainly to an extent that did not exist two decades ago.

Pfizer's bill for promoting Lyrica and other painkillers turned out to be a little higher than planned. A whole $2.3 billion higher. The company received the biggest criminal fine in US history when, in 2003, a sales rep turned whistle-blower accused Pfizer of promoting a painkiller (Bextra) for indications beyond its approval, and at doses that were too high and associated with serious side effects. The drug later had to be withdrawn because of safety concerns around cardiac and skin damage. A 2009 lawsuit saw Pfizer plead guilty to 'misbranding Bextra with the intent to defraud or mislead' and 'illegally promot[ing] four drugs'. One of the drugs included in the case was Lyrica. The prosecutor, Michael Loucks, described how doctors received generous kickbacks as part of the process: 'Pfizer invited [them] to consultant meetings, many in resort locations. Attendees' expenses were paid; they received a fee just for being there.' However, as *The New York Times* reported, the $2.3 billion fine amounted to 'less than three weeks of Pfizer's sales'.

The pharmaceutical industry's legacy as a player in the diagnostic elevation of fibromyalgia is undisputed, and its ability to mount similar battles undiminished. If the PAN/PANDAS community secures its interest, might a greater and more sustained acceptance follow – a symbiotic relationship of sorts?

The drugs being championed for the treatment of PANS and PANDAS target the immune system even though the role of autoimmunity is contested. Immunological markers have failed to correlate with clinical exacerbations in these patients, and autoantibody tests to differentiate between patients with PANDAS and control subjects have been inconsistent. But these failed correspondences haven't lowered the hopes of those who argue that steroids, intravenous immune globulin (IVIG) or plasma exchange (a dialysis-type procedure) could help. Also proposed are the same chemotherapy drugs used for cancer and in transplant patients to prevent organ rejection. It's an approach that, some argue, could rescue children from a horrible fate. In 2019, *Discover* magazine featured the case of Paul Michael, a 'quiet, brilliant kid you were likely to find in Silicon Valley − captivated by Lego, self-taught in origami, loving and sweet,' wrote journalist Pamela Weintraub. But at the age of seven, on 2 March 2009, he awoke 'monstrously changed'. He 'tore up the flooring in his bedroom. He got hold of a knife and stabbed holes through his door. He began speaking a strange language no one could understand. He tried pulling his teeth out. He barked like a dog.' He was diagnosed with PANS and treated for years with steroids, chemotherapy drugs and IVIG (as well as psychiatric therapy). In late 2013, Weintraub writes, 'sweet, smart Paul Michael, rescued by years of treatment, finally stepped out of the psych ward and back into his life. Today a gentle young man of 15, he goes to public school and hopes to be a pastry chef.'

However, in one 2016 trial, IVIG was not superior to a placebo. Other studies were partial in various ways: they did not include control or placebo groups, or were retrospective case reports or case series rather than randomised and blinded trials, or depended on subjective reports from parents rather than using formal assessment scales, or included children who were receiving other treatments (such as behavioural therapy and tic medications), making it difficult to assess the cause of any perceived benefit. Antibiotics treatment has failed to show any convincing effects, and its liberal use in some children has raised accusations of 'questionable antibiotic stewardship', which could cause lifelong antibiotic resistance and irreversible gut damage. Added to that, OCD and tic disorders follow a relapsing-remitting course, so any perceived benefit of treatment might in fact have little to do with that treatment, and instead simply reflect the natural history of how those symptoms might have resolved without any intervention.

There are two caveats to this rather gloomy view of PANS/PANDAS research. Firstly, the absence of evidence is disheartening, but does not rule out the potential that unbiased systematic research might provide enlightenment in the future. Secondly, it's easy to criticise immune treatments while disregarding the fact that the antipsychotics some of the children receive instead also carry significant long-term risks. 'I know the scientists want 7,000 controlled studies, double-blinded controlled trials,' says Georgia, 'but in the meantime these children and families are suffering, people have spent hundreds and thousands, they've lost everything. The power is in the hands of those who see the patients.'

Clinical trials will not prove whether or not PANS is 'real', as some observers hope. Such trials could, however, uncover which, if any, children with psychiatric symptoms benefit from antibiotics and immune treatments. It's likely that this group of children is a heterogeneous one. Some might have immune system dysfunction, and some might not. The dangers of treating all of them with the heavy-duty immunosuppressive regimens could be catastrophic. About 40% of all children receiving IVIG experience adverse effects; most are mild and transient – fatigue, chills, headache, abdominal pain and muscle aches, for instance – but 2–6% experience potentially serious reactions – blood clots, heart attacks, kidney failure, strokes and meningitis. It is irrefutable that most children given a diagnosis of PANDAS will not be harmed by IVIG, even if they are not helped by it. But it is not an exaggeration to say that lives are at stake here. The emotive discussion around miracle treatments must be countered by an acknowledgement of the potential perils of these treatments, and the risk of missing out on safe psychiatric care.

For the pharmaceutical industry, the yield could be high. Before them stand families who are desperate for treatments that happen to be expensive – thousands of pounds for a single infusion – and potentially lots of families: some advocates claim that PANS and PANDAS account for 10% of childhood-onset OCD and tic disorders. Susan Swedo estimates one in every 250–500 children develops the condition, and claims that around 1% of elementary school-aged children are affected. Some are willing to diagnose and treat many more: the New Jersey paediatric neurologist Rosario Trifiletti of the PANDAS/PANS Institute told *Cosmopolitan* magazine: 'There's probably one PANDAS kid in every kindergarten class.'

The families I spoke to have spent thousands of pounds on private medical consultations, international travel to meet with PANS and PANDAS specialists, and infusions for their children. They have maxed out credit cards and taken out loans. They are willing to do so again.

Harvey Singer, Professor of Neurology and Paediatrics at Johns Hopkins Hospital Children's Center in Baltimore, urges caution against unproven immune treatments: 'Until we fully understand this thing, our approach should be to treat symptoms. There are medicines that work with tics, so treat that. If they have OCD, there are medicines that treat that. If they have anxiety, we have drugs for that.' In another interview, he said: 'Parents like to have a simple explanation [...]. Sometimes what's simplest is not necessarily correct.'

The pharmaceutical industry breathed life into the diagnosis of fibromyalgia. If the industry sets its sights on the PANS and

PANDAS community, I imagine it will find people there who have felt rejected and scorned at times, ready to welcome its attentions.

Sometime this week, somewhere in the world, a parent will search online for an explanation of their child's tics and obsessions. They will find the acronym PANDAS, and they will meet other parents online who have travelled the same path – a community of kindred spirits. They will join other families consumed by a mission to ensure that PANS and PANDAS are understood and accepted; that their children's profound suffering is recognised in a way they believe does justice to them all.

Children like Finn and Lucas still need help and support, irrespective of whether they are deemed to have a physiological or psychiatric diagnosis. When it comes to these children's lives, the controversy over the authenticity of a diagnostic label threatens to overshadow their well-being. I hope that one day their recovery can transcend the diagnostic label.

7

An Abundance of Caution

It was 2012, and Abi was about to be tested for a mutation in a gene that had already left its mark across generations of her family. 'Cancer was coming down the tracks,' she says. 'My paternal grandmother had breast cancer at forty, then her daughter – my aunt – had it just before she turned forty. My sister had it at thirty-seven. And then a cousin had it at thirty-four.' Abi was thirty-two years old at the time. 'I'd just had my second child. He was two or three weeks old, and I got a phone call [telling me I had] a date to come in and meet the genetic counsellor,' Abi tells me. 'I remember looking down at my son in my arms and thinking, "What have I done to you? What if I passed this on to you as well?"'

She has another clear memory from the time – the genetic counsellor in Dublin walking into the clinic room with her results. 'The outside of the envelope was highlighted, and I said to myself, you're probably reading [too much] into this, but does that mean it's positive?'

Abi's suspicions were confirmed – she had a mutation of the BRCA1 gene. She had become, not quite someone with a diagnosis as we know it, but an inhabitant of the at-risk diagnostic space; a liminal zone somewhere between well and unwell.

Being a patient-in-waiting comes without the potentially grave consequences of full-blown disease, but also without any of the corollaries of having a categorically 'active' one – such as, perhaps,

201

due sympathy and consideration, sickness or disability payments, or a well-travelled roadmap for the treatment journey ahead. Speaking to cancer charities did not cross Abi's mind. 'I thought it [would be] wasteful of me, because there were people actually, genuinely really sick, who had lost a job because of their situation, and I didn't need to be taking up that time resource.'

A unifying and unavoidable message reaches all of those who exist in these ambiguous diagnostic spaces: 'Better safe than sorry.' They are urged, or feel compelled, to take action 'just in case'. Abi had to contend with life-changing decisions even as she was cancer-free. Should she have radical surgery to remove her breasts, even though they were healthy and might always be? Should she have her ovaries removed to reduce – but not eliminate – the risk of BRCA-related cancer, throwing her into premature menopause in her 30s? In this diagnostic waiting room, the medical prophet is fallible, the crystal ball obscured.

As I'll describe later in this chapter, the at-risk diagnostic land-scape even extends to the womb: to avoid their child being born with fetal alcohol syndrome, expectant women are instructed to abstain from alcohol – 'just in case'. Such a seemingly simple 'zero-alcohol' directive carries complex personal, ethical and even criminal ramifications for these women. I'll hear the story of Sean and James, young brothers from just outside Belfast, who were born with the syndrome and are living with its far-reaching consequences.

The state of being at risk: this is the new frontier of diagnosis. A land marked by lacunae of evidence and unreadable clouds, where sometimes making even an unwise decision feels better than making none. Our contemporary diagnoses reflect our overwhelming urge to minimise risk, or to eradicate it entirely – at an individual level, as with Abi's BRCA diagnosis; or at a societal one, as with fetal alcohol syndrome.

To understand this at-risk terrain, I first speak to Abi, who has spent years traversing her own diagnostic liminal space, created by the BRCA gene.

Breast cancer genes like BRCA1 and BRCA2 normally produce tumour suppressor proteins that help to repair DNA. With specific mutations in these genes, that repair process – a mechanism that protects against cancer – is impaired, and a normal cell can become a cancerous one.

Abi's initial session with her genetic counsellor mapped out what might lie ahead: 12% of women will develop breast cancer at some point during their lives, but 72% of women who inherit a harmful BRCA1 mutation will develop breast cancer by the age of 80. The risk of ovarian cancer with a BRCA1 mutation is 44% (this compares to 1.3% of women in the general population developing ovarian cancer at some point in their lives). BRCA mutations are also linked to fallopian tube, peritoneal and pancreatic cancer.

The BRCA at-risk journey is initially one of surveillance, with annual scans to detect cancer early on.* Abi felt for the most part that it was a chance to be proactive about her own well-being. 'Sometimes, though, I thought, "I don't have cancer. I shouldn't be clogging up waiting rooms, I shouldn't be taking up time on the MRI machine if I don't need it, I don't need to be costing the state a fortune."'

---

* Some opt for chemoprevention – drugs that reduce the risk of developing cancer. Its benefits are much clearer for BRCA2 than BRCA1 mutations, however. These drugs diminish the possibility of cancer rather than eradicate it, and can cause hot flushes, night sweats, vaginal discharge and dryness, and less commonly blood clots, cancer of the womb and strokes. Uptake remains low in the UK, as does awareness – less than one in seven women who are eligible for the treatment opt for it (see J. Hackett et al., 'Uptake of breast cancer preventive therapy in the UK', *Breast Cancer Research and Treatment*, 170/3 (2018)).

Soon, she was forced to confront the ineluctable dilemma faced by all patients with BRCA mutations: whether to choose drastic surgery over routine surveillance. Abi looked to her family history of cancer to make that call. Some have beaten the odds: 'My grandmother had survived to the age of eighty-something, a hale and hearty woman.' Her aunt had survived two rounds of breast cancer, and her own sister was now ten years cancer-free. But others had not been so lucky. Her cousin died 'a month shy of her fortieth birthday' some months ago – 'it's still very raw'. On the day she and I speak, her uncle is in a hospice, seeing out his last days. Men with BRCA mutations can also develop cancer – of the breast, prostate and pancreas.

Being at risk leads us towards treatment decisions that go beyond statistics; personal choices are shaped by intuition, and emotion. Some women with BRCA mutations are more likely to have risk-reducing surgery than others – those who have previously had breast cancer, those under the age of sixty, those who have already had children and, some studies suggest, those who have watched close family members experience cancer, especially a mother or sister. Financial pressures and access to healthcare inform these choices too.*

Abi, who was perfectly well by all the traditional measures we

---

* Rates also vary between nations. In one study of ten countries, they were highest in the US (around 50%) and lowest in Poland (4.5%) (K. Metcalfe et al., 'International trends in the uptake of cancer risk reduction strategies in women with a *BRCA1* or *BRCA2* mutation', *British Journal of Cancer*, 121 (2019)). The UK was not included in this study, but trends suggest that patients are increasingly choosing risk-reducing surgery over surveillance screening only. Demand for BRCA1/2 testing almost doubled here after actor Angelina Jolie announced her positive BRCA status and subsequent surgery. Researchers have reported a 2.5-fold increase in uptake of bilateral mastectomy in the two years following her revelation.

use to determine health, chose the sort of extensive surgery usually reserved for those with advanced cancer. Until now, her body had borne no signs of the genetic anomaly she had inherited. Soon, the scars of surgery would leave their imprint in perpetuity.

On St Valentine's Day 2014, aged thirty-four and then a mother of three children under five, Abi had a bilateral mastectomy. That surgery reduced her risk of breast cancer by at least 95%, to even less than that in women without a genetic mutation. But the procedure was marred by a series of brutal complications, including infections and necrosis:

> I was supposed to have one surgery. It turned into seven.
> Afterwards, for that two-and-a-half-year period, I was
> wrecked, absolutely wrecked, and I wasn't in a good
> place. I was just trying to get my strength back to go
> again for another surgery, which I knew was going to
> actually be the hardest one.

That next surgery was a bilateral salpingo-oophorectomy (BSO) – removal of the ovaries and fallopian tubes. BSO dramatically decreases the chances of cancer, but it carries the risk of premature menopause (which in turn can be associated with cardiovascular disease and osteoporosis) and affects fertility.* The clock was ticking for Abi; the risk of ovarian cancer rises in a woman's early to mid-forties. She underwent BSO surgery in 2017, when her

---

* Having both surgeries – bilateral mastectomy and BSO – results in an 80% reduction of risk of dying from ovarian cancer, according to a study of almost 2,500 women in Europe and North America (Susan M. Domchek et al., 'Association of Risk-Reducing Surgery in BRCA1 or BRCA2 Mutation Carriers with Cancer Risk and Mortality', *JAMA*, 304/9 (2010)). The surgeries are not failsafe, however. Tissue can remain behind where cancer will develop, and cancer can still develop elsewhere.

third son was nine months old. Once again, her post-operative course was stormy: 'Everything from dry eyeballs to being really cranky and cross and angry at the world, ups and downs with your mental health [...] you know with the drop in hormones, you really become a whole different person and nothing can prepare you for it.' HRT, time and tremendous support from her family helped her to pull through. 'It's only looking at us now, here and now, you kind of see how that just didn't affect me, it affected everybody.'

The familial legacy of BRCA still weighs on her mind. In her family of five siblings, three have tested positive – including herself. There's the next generation to think of too. 'My eldest is twelve and for the very first time, last weekend, we started to have the conversation.' After her uncle was admitted to a hospice, her son asked, 'Why do so many people in your family have cancer?' Abi answered in the best way she could for now.

> I said to him, 'We do have a risk in our family. Do
> you remember when you were small, and I was in the
> hospital a little bit? I was doing things to make sure that
> I wasn't going to get cancer. Isn't that great, that I could
> do that? Now I'm not going to get cancer, most likely.'

Each of her children has a 50% chance of inheriting a BRCA mutation. They may choose to undergo genetic testing at the age of eighteen (deemed the legal age of consent for this sort of testing), but there will be more complex conversations ahead. Abi is taking it one step at a time.

When she left her genetic counselling appointment in 2012, there was little follow-up support. 'All I had was a photocopy of my results and this Post-it note that gave you a few websites to look at.' Now, as one of a team of BRCA-positive peer support volunteers for a cancer charity, she aims to provide solace to those embarking on the same journey. 'We talk too about how you engage with the rest of the family, because you're on a completely different trajectory. People feel, not left behind, but … it's a very strange space, how do you come together after something like that? A line has divided your family.'

Despite the arduous journey she has been on – repeated surgeries with their unremitting complications, all of those psychological and physical scars – Abi advocates access to BRCA testing in those whose family history suggests they are at high risk, while supporting people's choice not to be tested after genetic counselling:

> People should be offered the opportunities to stay in the
> lives of their loved ones, to walk up the aisle, to grow
> old with their partner. It's very empowering to have that
> information. I suppose that's one of the messages I want
> to convey: that there is this fantastic opportunity, it's not
> all negative, it's an opportunity to live your life without
> worry […] This is in your hands, it's about what you
> want to do with it.

The envelope that held Abi's genetic results had been highlighted. It could not bring certainty, but it did provide a clear demarcation from normality; the report in that envelope left her with statistics to work with, figures to guide her decision. It was a call to action.

But what if the envelope only carries shades of grey? What then?

In your shades-of-grey envelope, you'll increasingly see this acronym: VUS. 'Variants of unknown significance' are indeterminate genetic mutations that reflect a change to the expected genetic code. But it's a vague finding, because it hasn't been seen with any frequency in the testing laboratory and hasn't been classed as *not* causing disease, to date at least. It's difficult to know what to do with a VUS – it's not positive, it's not negative, it could be harmless, but it might not be. Almost a fifth of patients with cancer who undergo genetic testing learn they have a VUS. Close to 30% of patients tested for gene mutations related to heart disease receive the same news. Ethnic minority populations are even more likely to be presented with a VUS result: public databases and many laboratories carry a greater proportion of genetic results from white people, which means that a genetic variant which exists in a person from a 'non-white' background will more often be deemed rare and thus considered a VUS.

Our capacity to sequence our genes has outpaced our understanding of the landscape. Direct-to-consumer genetic testing kits are landing on our doorsteps each day, with the global market forecast to reach $6.36 billion by 2028. Through these kits, more of us are bypassing the prevailing strict criteria for screening in medicine, which is typically limited to those with a strong family history of early-onset disease. These commercial companies usually test for genetic variants (not actual disease-causing mutations) associated with an increased risk of conditions such as chronic kidney disease, Parkinson's, late-onset Alzheimer's dementia, coeliac disease and age-related macular degeneration, among others. But many of these diseases have been primarily and more convincingly linked to environmental influences – diet and smoking, for instance – rather than purely genetic ones; or at least, there's a complex interaction between the two. You might need to inherit several other variants (which are not tested for) for a disorder to make itself known, and there's rarely, if ever, any reassuring information on the variants that *reduce* your risk of a disease. The number of available tests is only rivalled by the number of disclaimer forms that accompany them.

Your chance of being genetically tested as a hospital patient has risen too, with the remarkable expansion of techniques that rapidly and cheaply sequence numerous genes at a time. At least five million NHS patients will be tested for gene mutations for rare diseases and cancer by 2024, in a process that is being embedded into routine clinical care. This project could yield a transformative understanding of these conditions, and it reassuringly examines the whole genome rather than performs a selective analysis of short stretches of DNA (which is what some commercial companies do – the equivalent of a very selective subeditor); and patients receive specific genetic counselling about the possibility of receiving a VUS result.*

But elsewhere, the ambiguity conferred by a VUS propels not cautious responses, but extreme ones. Guidelines warn against using VUSs in isolation to make clinical decisions, but up to half of surgeons in one US study took the same management decisions for their patients – frequently a bilateral mastectomy – regardless of whether their patients had a VUS or a clearly disease-causing BRCA mutation.

Patients may also grasp for certainty in a sea of confusion. Eighty per cent of women with variants of unknown significance interpreted these findings as showing a genetic predisposition

---

* About 1 in 100 participants in the UK's 100,000 Genomes Project is expected to learn of additional genetic abnormalities unrelated to the cancer or rare disease that prompted them to take part in the first place, including 'at risk' genetic mutations for bowel, breast and ovarian cancers, and familial hypercholesterolaemia. For now, researchers only search for these additional abnormalities with a patient's consent and state that 'people who consented to this analysis are only informed where there is strong scientific evidence that the changes in their genome can cause a disease'. See Genomics England, 'Information for 100,000 Genomes Project participants: additional findings', https://www.genomicsengland.co.uk.

for cancer, and over half of those who interpreted the results as potentially disease-causing had surgery to decrease their risk. In fact, almost the same number of women with an indeterminate result opted for surgery as those with a clearly pathogenic (disease-causing) mutation. Most of them distinctly remembered being told that the result was non-informative, and yet still interpreted it as putting them at risk of cancer. Why this reaction? In making their decision, some patients privileged memories of loved ones experiencing cancer over the test result alone. Others may have sought a sense of control, researchers speculate, by 'transforming the gray color of the DNA-test result into black or white'.

The international ENIGMA Consortium is working to bring lucidity to the abstruse world of the VUS – this collaborative network of scientists has collected thousands of these variants across seventeen countries, in a Holmesian bid to decipher them – but there are still no internationally accepted standards for how these tests are reported and no agreed consistent classification system.

Knowing your genetic blueprint could steer you towards pre-emptive action to protect your health, it could inform the life you live now or the decisions you make for your family's future. But each time we determine risk in medicine, although we search for clarity, we may instead be overwhelmed by confusion. The ostensibly well suddenly become patients.

In the diagnostic world of VUSs, the 'better safe than sorry' message seems inadequate. You are challenged to act based on highly ambiguous data. Should you tell your children about a gene they may or may not inherit, one that may or may not impact them? Should you have radical surgery to prevent a condition that has little chance of emerging? With time, scientists may escalate your variant to 'pathogenic' or de-prioritise it to 'benign', but by that time you may have already made your irreversible decision.

These are the complexities of managing risk in medicine. But for those opportunities when definitive steps *can* be taken and the evidence base at least offers more robust support – screening to catch BRCA-related cancer early, or surgery to try and prevent it entirely – uncertainty is the price we might have to pay. Abi's story speaks to this. She has somehow grasped hold of the ambiguity and taken action to reduce her risk, and her children can do so too. Sometimes, the diagnostic liminal space, despite its challenges, is worth visiting.

There is another diagnosis that provokes us to consider the question of risk, and how we unravel it in medicine. The diagnosis itself – fetal alcohol syndrome – is not in question, but the measures mothers are told to take to avoid it are. What do we gain or lose when we aim for zero risk, and who pays the price?

'They know that they have a tummy mummy. And tummy mummy drank alcohol when they were in her tummy.' That's how Alison explains their situation to Sean, aged thirteen, and James, aged twelve. 'I tell them alcohol made their brains different, so they learn different. But it also makes them very special.'

Fetal alcohol syndrome (FAS) was first described in 1973 by a group of Seattle researchers. They wrote about three affected babies born to 'American Indian chronic alcoholic mothers'. Heavy drinking was so dangerous for developing babies, they explained in the *Lancet*, that 'serious consideration should be given toward early termination of pregnancy in such women'.

More than three decades later in Cumbria, Alison and her husband Brian adopted 23-month-old Sean; his brother James came into their lives several months later. The clues that something was amiss emerged quickly. The brothers were not hitting their developmental milestones, mealtimes at nursery were especially fraught, and intense temper tantrums were commonplace. Traces of the cause could be seen in their distinct physical appearance. 'This guardian came up to our house and she took one look at James and said, "Has anyone ever talked to you about fetal alcohol syndrome?"' It immediately made sense to Alison. 'I knew the lifestyle that [their] birth mummy had lived,' she tells me. It might escape notice at first glance, but Sean and James (not their real names) have the syndrome's typical facial features – a thin upper lip and a flattening of the philtrum, the vertical groove between the nose and upper lip. Babies born with FAS have restricted growth and tend to be shorter than their peers throughout their lives. Some children, like James, have smaller heads and many have short palpebral fissures (narrowed eye openings).

The family soon moved to Northern Ireland – they now live in a village 20 miles outside Belfast. At school, the impact of alcohol on the boys' brain development became obvious. Children with FAS have intellectual delay, communication difficulties and impaired fine motor skills. Memory issues are characteristic – 'For Sean, when he goes to the shop, if it's more than three things I have to write them on a piece of paper for him. For James, we're lucky if he can remember one or two' – as is impairment in language, mental processing, problem solving, judgement and reasoning. 'Sean is now reading at his age level, but it's taken a lot of work with him. James can't read or write properly. He's twelve. We're still very much [at] basic preschool age.'

Some children with FAS have attention deficit or hyperactivity with obsessional behaviours, poor impulse control and impaired social skills that endure into adulthood. 'We call it Groundhog Day,' Alison explains:

> We have to do things by a certain routine, otherwise
> it throws them off. There are meltdowns – like the
> tantrums of a two-year-old, at the zoo, on the ferry,

at the shops – and people, they look at you like you're
something underneath their foot. Then they look at
the child, and they're like, 'How can any child behave
like that?'

Following a series of visits to paediatricians and geneticists, James
was confirmed as having FASD – fetal alcohol spectrum disorder,
an umbrella term that includes the full-blown presentation
of FAS alongside partial forms that show some, but not all, its
clinical features. For Sean, the diagnostic conclusion was 'features
associated with FASD'. There were additional circumstances
related to his birth – beyond alcohol – which doctors believe
could have contributed to his cognitive and behavioural issues.

In the 1970s – the time of that original Seattle FAS study –
as easy as it was to find evidence that sustained heavy drinking
and binge drinking could affect the fetus, what constituted a 'safe'
amount of alcohol was unclear. Nevertheless, in 1981 the acting
US Surgeon General Edward Brandt advised women who were
pregnant or considering pregnancy not to drink alcohol, even
though FAS case reports at the time described the syndrome in
babies born to mothers who drank 'a bottle of liquor a day', '20
drinks a day', '1.5 quarts of beer per day for 7 years', 'a gallon of
wine and a half case of beer every Friday and Saturday evening' and
'three to four pints of liquor a day'. The link between alcohol and
FAS was not linear – up to 95% of women who drank heavily did
not give birth to children with the syndrome. Additional factors
primed the development of FAS, researchers proposed, including
malnourishment, smoking and stress, which triggered cellular
changes in some drinkers that, in turn, enhanced the toxicity of
alcohol. Reducing the syndrome to purely a matter of maternal
personal choice seemed to overlook mothers' lived circumstances
and social disadvantages.

Brandt's 1981 advice still reverberates today. In 2016, Professor Dame Sally Davies, then Chief Medical Officer for England, said:

> I want pregnant women to be very clear that they
> should avoid alcohol as a precaution. Although the risk
> of harm to the baby is low if they have drunk small
> amounts of alcohol before becoming aware of the
> pregnancy, there is no 'safe' level of alcohol to drink
> when you are pregnant.*

The CDC goes one step further, instructing all sexually active women of reproductive age who are not using birth control to abstain completely from alcohol, even if they are not trying to conceive. They defend this edict on the basis that many pregnancies are unplanned, and most women do not know they are pregnant until four to six weeks in. In 2020, the WHO released its draft Global Alcohol Action Plan, which states that 'appropriate attention [...] should be given to prevention of drinking among pregnant women and women of childbearing age'. Despite these warnings, drinking during pregnancy is not exceptional. Between 40% and 80% of women drink in pregnancy in the UK, Ireland, Australia and New Zealand, and the WHO reports the global prevalence of alcohol use in pregnancy as 9.8%, with the highest

---

* Starting in 2016, the UK Department of Health and Social Care had advised pregnant women who chose to drink to limit their alcohol intake to 'no more than 1 to 2 units of alcohol once or twice per week'. The Royal College of Obstetricians and Gynaecologists (RCOG) now advises total abstinence to pregnant women, having previously (in 2013) issued advice to 'not drink more than one or two units, and then not more than once or twice a week' (see RCOG, 'RCOG statement on BJOG study that suggests light drinking in pregnancy is not linked to developmental problems in childhood', 17 April 2013).

rates in Russia (36.5%) and the UK (41.3%).* Many women stop drinking once they learn that they are expecting – in 7,000 New Zealand women, 71% drank alcohol in the first trimester, but 43% stopped when they discovered they were pregnant.

Sean and James's experiences underscore the devastating toll of fetal alcohol syndrome. They are not alone: worldwide, around 119,000 children are born each year with FAS – and the figure for FASD is believed to be much higher.† Even this basic discernment of FAS is fraught with difficulty. Accurate and consistent figures are difficult to ascertain because of both a failure to recognise the condition, and an over-recognition in populations perceived to be high-risk, i.e. minorities, and children in care or in the correctional system. There are wide variations in study methodology, no single FAS classification system, and no routine collection of FAS data in the UK. Even if a child has the typical physical and cognitive features and their mother drank high volumes of alcohol in pregnancy, no test can prove an irrefutable causal link.

So in this terrain of things unknown, we grasp for one thing that seems certain: heavy alcohol use is a known and preventable cause of birth defects, and can cause stillbirths and miscarriages. If FAS is predictable and preventable, aren't we obliged to ensure that no child is ever put at risk of developing it?

The zero-tolerance alcohol approach – even for women

---

* The wide range in estimated rates between countries and between studies may partly be down to the different research methods used, particularly since some studies ask women about their drinking at antenatal clinic interviews – an environment where they might be reluctant to disclose this information – while others calculate numbers though anonymised surveys.

† The CDC estimates that 0.2 to 1.5 infants are born with FAS for every 1,000 live births in Alaska, Arizona, Colorado and New York. The WHO estimates that 15 in every 10,000 people globally have FAS.

not planning to conceive – has thrived. Isn't it worth simply foregoing a couple of glasses of wine a week, most public health campaigners ask, to ensure the well-being of one's child? A moral obligation worth fulfilling, a small surrender; perhaps even one that satisfies the widespread cultural expectation of self-sacrifice in motherhood. Through abstinence the risk to a baby is eliminated, seemingly without any truly harmful lasting consequence for these women.

Yet there is a wider conversation to be had, one that perhaps requires a little more nuance. We must hold in our minds Sean and James, and the high price they have paid, but it's worth exploring – without fear of censure – the deeper questions that the diagnosis of FAS touches on: about how we approach risk in medicine, and what happens when we try to eliminate it.

So let's try asking the question again: in pregnancy, how much alcohol is too much? The one sort of trial that might provide an answer is a randomised one, where researchers assign alcohol (low and high volumes) to one group of pregnant women while telling another group to abstain, before eventually assessing their babies over time, with physical and cognitive tests. This sort of unethical trial will justifiably never come to pass. Instead, researchers draw on the self-reports of women who choose to drink during pregnancy (or drank before realising they were pregnant), and then relate these findings to fetal and childhood outcomes.

Researchers in Bristol recently analysed twenty-six studies, and made a simple assertion in the *BMJ*: it is not possible to say that light amounts of alcohol consumption harm a developing fetus. They defined this light amount as up to two UK units of alcohol up to twice a week – that is, a total of 4 units spread over the week, rather than all in one go. That equates to a little over a pint of high-strength (5.2%) beer, lager or cider, or two 175ml glasses of (12%) wine a week. Sounding a cautionary note, however, they acknowledged that the absence of evidence (for harm to the fetus) does not equate to evidence of absence.

The responses to these findings among the scientific community appeared contradictory. Sir David Spiegelhalter, Professor of the Public Understanding of Risk at the University of Cambridge, said that 'this valuable and humane study has shown that warnings about the dangers of drinking any alcohol at all during pregnancy are not justified by evidence'; while Professor Russell Viner, formerly Officer for Health Promotion at the Royal College of Paediatrics and Child Health, took a different line: 'My advice to women is that it's best not to drink at all if you're trying for a baby or pregnant. Regularly drinking even small amounts could be harmful and should be avoided, in line with the precautionary approach.'

The precautionary principle regarding abstinence is broadly one of 'better safe than sorry, even if the chance of harm is remote'. The principle came to prominence in the 1980s, when it was leveraged to justify vigorous environmental policies to tackle acid rain, global warming and pollution in West Germany.

An influential definition emerged in the Rio Declaration on Environment and Development in 1992: 'Where there are threats of serious or irreversible damage, lack of full scientific certainty shall not be used as a reason for postponing cost-effective measures to prevent environmental degradation'. Proponents of the precautionary principle argue that in the past, waiting for proof of causal relationships – for example, between asbestos and lung cancer, or lead exposure and brain damage in children – meant that the chance to avert harm was tragically lost. And so, they argue, when a potential outcome is catastrophic, mitigating action must be taken to prevent damage, even in the absence of equivocal scientific evidence to guide this action. The precautionary

principle has now been introduced to the sphere of public health
– it acts as a response to uncertainty and is driven primarily by
fear of the future over evidence from the past, and in the case
of FAS it has led to an edict on abstinence. This has striking
ethical and societal consequences that traditional, uncontested
risk-reduction strategies in individual patients (taking a blood
pressure tablet to reduce one's chance of stroke, for instance) do
not. Pregnant women who choose to drink – even lightly – come
under suspicion of being reckless regarding their baby's health,
despite the absence of evidence of harm. We've all heard stories
of pregnant women being refused service in a bar or restaurant
(or at least accounts of their drink being served with a garnish
of judgement and moral rectitude). Value-laden, even puritanical,
national campaigns flourish. A German Brewers' Association
campaign claimed that 'every sip of alcohol during pregnancy can
severely affect the health of an unborn child'. A similar initiative
in the Ukraine was called 'The "Virgin" Pregnancy' campaign, and
an Italian campaign showed a fetus in a cocktail glass, submerged
under alcohol, ice cubes and a slice of orange: '*Mama Beve, Bimbo
Beve*' – '[When] Mother Drinks, Baby Drinks'. The advertisement
appeared in bars, restaurants and toilet cubicles, and on buses.

If you have a drink in Moldova or Turkey, you'll find a
pregnancy warning on the bottle: a silhouette of a pregnant
woman, drink in hand, a diagonal red line emblazoned across her
body. Similar signage is becoming increasingly common, though
not yet mandatory, on bottles in the UK. Around 30 countries
legally require pregnancy warning labels on alcoholic drinks,
including France, Mexico, Lithuania, South Africa, Russia, the
US and, most recently, Australia and New Zealand. Studies show
that these labels do not influence average consumption or incite
behavioural change, and warnings are rarely noticed in the UK
– have a look next time you open a bottle of wine – although

proponents of this sort of signage are pushing for it to be given greater prominence.

I sense echoes here of the long-standing medical practice of implicating mothers or mothers-to-be in harm that comes to their children, and of a deep-rooted cultural desire to distinguish 'bad' mothers from 'good' ones, 'responsible' ones from 'irresponsible' ones, and 'self-indulgent', 'sybaritic', 'selfish' ones from 'self-sacrificing', 'nurturing' ones. In the 1930s and 1940s, 'schizophrenogenic mothers' – supposedly remote, rigid and unemotional – were blamed, without warrant, for their child's mental illness. In the 1950s, some omniscient psychoanalysts described 'refrigerator mothers' – seemingly defective women whose emotional detachment and frigidity directly contaminated their children, leading to autism. While some mothers were too ambivalent, others were not ambivalent enough. Dr Edward Strecker, a former president of the APA, said that overprotective mothers had 'failed in the elementary mother function of weaning [their] offspring emotionally as well as physically'. Strecker served as special consultant to the Secretary of War and the Secretary of the Navy, and believed that the mothers who instilled 'neurosis and weakness' in their sons during wartime were 'our gravest menace, a threat to our survival'. It would seem remiss to imagine that some of these contested discussions around FAS are unspoilt by an entrenched cultural ideology of motherhood.

Today's alcohol advice to pregnant women privileges the precautionary principle over conventional risk management that is grounded in evidence regarding both probability and outcomes. 'What to avoid in pregnancy' lists are lengthy: leading go-to patient websites warn women against too much sunbathing, too much caffeine, too much sugar, too much hair dye, too much sitting (but beware of too much exercise) and too high a heel. In the last ten years, a vogue for maternal genetics has taken hold: 'Mother's diet during pregnancy alters baby's DNA' (BBC News, 18 April 2011) and 'Pregnant 9/11 survivors transmitted trauma to their children' (*Guardian*, 9 September 2011). Irrespective of how real or speculative or wholly nonsensical these perceived risks are, the lack of specificity and nuance around these warnings leave many pregnant women feeling stressed or punished, and wondering what, if any, medical advice they should engage with.

The role of fathers usually passes without comment. Some, but by no means all, animal studies have suggested that paternal alcohol consumption before conception causes signs of brain impairment including stunted growth, hyperactivity, impaired learning and incoordination in mice offspring. A recent Norwegian study of (human) couples reported higher odds of microcephaly – smaller head circumference, a marker for brain development – at birth for higher paternal alcohol consumption before pregnancy. There is no consensus on whether paternal intake of alcohol can lead to fetal alcohol syndrome, not helped by the fact the question has rarely been researched.

As for FAS, this is tricky ethical territory, the ethicist Dr Julian Sheather acknowledges in a BMA report. It is not that a pregnant woman owes *no* duties of any kind to a fetus she wishes to carry to term, he writes, but these duties are not enforceable, since 'any move toward conferring legal rights on fetuses that are enforceable against the pregnant woman would have significant repercussions'. We are obliged to contemplate whether such a move could undermine existing rights for women to seek an abortion, for instance, and where such coercive measures might end. He encourages us, in answering these questions he poses, to think about 'whether incarceration would be considered for pregnant women who put their fetus at risk in other ways, by involvement in extreme sports or continuing in high-risk occupations'.

Conversely, a joint team from the University of Oxford and

Melbourne Law School has argued that there *is* an ethical and legal case for intervening to prevent serious harm to a future child, 'even if the fetus is regarded as having no legal or moral status'. Writing in the *Bioethics* journal, they identify potential schemes to achieve this – voluntary counselling for pregnant women about 'safe levels of alcohol intake', or programmes that target pregnant women who drink heavily. These are relatively small infringements of a women's autonomy, they believe: 'Where it is possible to avert harm by taking actions that involve little or no self-sacrifice, the Duty of Easy Rescue implies that there is a strong ethical obligation to take that action'. They also, more controversially, explore harsher interventions: restricting the serving or selling of alcohol to pregnant women; mandatory reporting of pregnant women believed to be risking their future child's welfare; and mandatory counselling for pregnant women with a history of 'risky drinking'. These measures should be adopted to prevent future harm, they contend, since 'the harm to the pregnant woman imposed by [these] interventions may seem to be vastly outweighed by the potential harm to the future child that is prevented'.

The reality is inevitably much more complex. Several US states support mandatory reporting of women's behaviours during pregnancy to law enforcement or child welfare agencies. The use of intoxicants in pregnancy is legally classified as child abuse or neglect in twenty states. A diagnosis of FAS after birth is not required. In Arizona, mandatory reporting to child services is indicated for a newborn who 'may be affected by the presence of alcohol'. In Minnesota, reporting to a welfare agency is required by law if there is a 'reason to believe' that a pregnant woman 'has consumed alcoholic beverages during the pregnancy in any way that is habitual or excessive'.

In states that have policies that target alcohol use during pregnancy, more babies are born prematurely and with low birthweight, research shows. It's a finding that might seem paradoxical at first, but if pregnant women think they are drinking more than they should, they may be reticent to seek prenatal care more broadly, as well as alcohol-specific counselling or rehabilitation. Women have frequently faced involuntary treatment, protective custody and jail time, and have had their children removed by child protective services – irrespective of whether their child has come to harm.

A 2011 study from the University of California, Berkeley showed the potentially corrosive and discriminatory nature of these judgements: black women are more likely to be screened for alcohol and drug use in prenatal care, even though they are only as likely to be identified as having alcohol or drug use issues during pregnancy as white women. Black women are more likely than others to face legal consequences for prenatal drug use. Black newborns are four times more likely than white newborns to be reported to child protective services at delivery, even when their mothers have already received treatment for their alcohol or drug use. Black women are more likely to lose custody of their child as a result, and less likely to be reunited with them. There are similar findings for poor pregnant women, ethnic minority or not, who are disproportionately tested for drugs and more likely to be reported to health and child welfare authorities, even when their alcohol use parallels that of white middle-class women.

Pregnant women in the UK do not face these sorts of legal threats, but they are not free from scrutiny. In England and Wales, plans were announced in 2020 for a consultation on whether or not to record the alcohol intake of all expectant mothers, prompting concerns about overreach and data privacy. The proposed changes would mean that a single drink taken by a woman before she was aware that she was pregnant would be documented, and this information would be transferred from her own antenatal record to her baby's, without maternal consent being required, and out of step with usual patient confidentiality practices. This is already established practice in a number of health trusts, including one in Manchester, where midwives use 'demonstration FASD dolls' with facial malformation to warn women of the impact of alcohol. The drinking habits of fathers-to-be are not documented.

The truth is that calculating the risk of a diagnosis of FAS, and calculating risk in medicine more broadly, creates a tension in which 'zero tolerance' prevails. The BMA explains its stance on abstinence in pregnancy by citing three factors: the widespread variation in emphasis in guidance and advice, compounded by confusing and conflicting media reports; the misinterpretation of guidelines and limits, as 'individuals may not clearly understand what units or "standard drinks" are'; and the ineffectiveness of providing information on standard alcohol measures which '[do] not appear to prevent [people] consuming more than they realise': 'Taking these factors into consideration, the BMA believes that, on balance, the safest approach is for women who are pregnant, or who are considering a pregnancy, to be advised not to consume any alcohol.' The judgement is therefore not based on unequivocal science, as the report carefully acknowledges, but instead the only route the organisation (and many others) can conscionably find to provide, in their words, 'a clear, unequivocal public health message'.

Some mainstream websites for pregnant women are less nuanced in their messaging.

BabyCentre UK states that 'it's especially important to steer clear of alcohol in the first trimester […]. Too much alcohol can permanently damage your developing baby's cells. Your baby's face, organs and brain might not grow properly'. The independent UK alcohol education charity Drinkaware states: 'Most importantly, stop drinking as soon as you do realise you're pregnant.' The National Childbirth Trust (NCT) poses the question whether it is 'safe to drink a little during pregnancy'. Its answer: 'The advice is – no, not really.' The NHS start4life website states that 'it's safer not to drink alcohol during pregnancy, or if you are planning to become pregnant, because it can damage your growing baby. By not drinking, you are protecting your baby and minimising the risks to their development and future health'.

There is a failure, then, to acknowledge that there is no unequivocal evidence that low levels of alcohol consumption do harm to a baby. Does society think that pregnant women cannot process a message that goes beyond 'this is for your baby's good'? Is there no case for openly stating that binge drinking and heavy drinking may irrevocably harm a fetus, but that science does not provide the same indisputable link for light drinking? Public health and media organisations have the capacity to elevate the subtlety, sensitivity and quality of their messaging, rather than issuing seemingly axiomatic abstinence directives that abdicate their own responsibility to communicate clearly.

Throughout this book, we've seen a pattern emerge, one of which FAS is a part: external stakeholders influence who gets to make a diagnosis, how it is used and how it is policed.

Exploring these complexities can produce understandably impassioned yet thoughtful responses, but sometimes also incur unadulterated wrath and opprobrium. In 2013, the economics professor and author Emily Oster wrote *Expecting Better: Why the Conventional Pregnancy Wisdom is Wrong and What You Really Need to Know*, which included a section on FAS. The National Organization on Fetal Alcohol Syndrome (NOFAS) issued a press release, calling her book 'flawed and harmful', and stated that 'if Emily Oster is willing to tolerate the risk, that's her choice, but it's irresponsible to encourage other pregnant women to take the risk with their children'. NOFAS posted an article she had written on FAS on its Facebook page, with a request to their followers to 'please leave a review of her harmful book on

Amazon'. Commentators wrote that she should spend time with children with FAS, labelled her an 'idiot' and an 'arrogant ass', and proposed a petition to have the book removed, and a boycott of the book's publisher.

When I think of Sean and James, I can understand the emotional responses to any questioning of the abstinence message. The brothers undeniably have a difficult journey ahead. 'The future scares the living daylights out of me, because I worry what will happen to them,' their mother Alison says. She is all too aware that children with FAS are more likely to develop lifelong psychiatric and academic issues, fall into substance misuse and experience run-ins with the law.

She takes comfort from their many strengths, though. 'Sean has got one of the most amazing imaginations I've ever come across in a child. He can watch something, and then he can act it out. James is football-mad. That boy cannot read or write but he knows every Liverpool player, he knows the numbers on their shirts.' She is proud of their generosity too:

> The two of them arranged for a bouquet of flowers to
> be delivered to me this Mother's Day. From their own
> birthday money, bless them. Even my husband didn't
> know that they done it. You know, they will never leave
> anybody out. They've got the biggest hearts of any
> children I've ever come across. I'm not just saying that
> because they're my sons.

She has established a non-profit group for FASD in Northern Ireland offering support to other families affected by the condition. She also provides training for midwives. Her stance is unambiguous. 'There's no middle ground. If you drink whilst you're pregnant, you're playing Russian roulette with that baby's life. The rule of thumb is "don't drink". If you're thinking of becoming pregnant, both you and your partner need to cut out the alcohol.'

It's a message that, as an influential figure in her local FASD community, she is keen to share. 'It needs to be part of the school syllabus. When I worked in boarding schools, we covered sex, drugs and rock and roll, but not what alcohol does.' She is pushing health authorities to expand their involvement too. 'You go into the hospitals or paediatric units [and] there are posters there – "Don't smoke while you're pregnant" and "Don't take drugs". There is nothing [saying] "Don't drink".' She draws the line, though, at mandatory bans on drinking during pregnancy: 'It would just cause an uproar.'

Alison asks me to convey a message about her, her husband and her organisation. 'We are non-judgemental. You know, [a young girl has a] one-night stand and she's ended up falling pregnant. Or she [...] might not even know that she's pregnant for the first few months, and she's still out there drinking – we don't judge that at all, we're just here to say, "Look, this is what can happen." We just want them to know that we're here if they need help and advice. We're here for people who have got fetal alcohol children.'

Calculating and managing risk in medicine is complicated. Abi's story speaks to the space it offers for empowerment, the chance to be proactive, even the prospect of recasting one's future. But with more opaque genetic findings such as the VUS, the idea that 'forewarned is forearmed' becomes more contentious – such knowledge may only hang over us like a sword of Damocles. FAS is emblematic of how we cope with extreme uncertainty in medicine. There, the precautionary principle is an alluring one – minor acts of self-sacrifice appear to be desirable for the greater good. But if the aim of the precautionary principle is to do no harm, here it falls short of that aspiration. Minimising and eliminating risk have ethical and actual ramifications, especially in groups that are already marginalised. The paternalistic old days of medicine saw some doctors, at least, make unilateral decisions with little patient consultation, withholding their knowledge of alternative options, side effects and risks from patients 'for their own good'. This resonates in some of our liminal diagnoses today – frequently championed by those far from the medical front line. In the hinterland of the at-risk diagnosis, we have the chance to reset the narrative of paternalism. Let this opportunity not be lost.

Epilogue

My uncle was a family doctor in Shillong, a hill station in north-eastern India. Shillong sits at 6,500 feet, enveloped by clouds, cloaked in blue Vanda orchids, cobra lilies and gnarled crepe myrtle trees with orange and scarlet leaves. In the evenings, on the veranda under a magnolia tree, my uncle would tell me stories of the patients who came to him from the villages. The parents who believed their child's squint was a blessing – Lakshmi, the goddess of wealth and prosperity, had one just like it. And the locals who described measles as *Ai* ('mother'): a measles rash announced the arrival of a Hindu mother goddess, and so, the belief went, the sick child was to be worshipped and bestowed with their choice of gifts. When his sister, my aunt, developed measles as a child, her family understood it to be an infection. But they also hoped to fulfil her wish: that of a white flower. My grandfather brought home a magnolia shrub, the closest thing he could find that day. It grew into the tree that now towered over us.

Diagnoses are best understood locally, then, in dialects and idioms and vernaculars. They are a matter of context; however much we might wish it, they do not have consistency or uniformity across time and place. We have seen how their fluidity is not inevitably a shortcoming, but it does mean they are exquisitely sensitive to external forces – moral, political, cultural. The very impartiality of our diagnoses compels us to hold them up to the light, admit to their imperfections, and strive to repair the damage that we see. It would be a mistake to believe that this sensitivity is limited to psychiatric diagnoses. Consider the disciplines that cross paths with the conditions we have met in this book: excited delirium (forensic pathology), status lymphaticus (paediatrics, anaesthetics, pathology), PANDAS (immunology, neurology), fetal alcohol syndrome (obstetrics, paediatrics, public health) and spermatorrhea (surgery).

There's no question that diagnostic labels have the capacity to direct us towards cure and consideration. In Ayesha's case, a PTSD diagnosis offered the tantalising possibility of removing her to a place of safety after perilous and damaging months spent in a refugee camp. But at their worst, diagnoses make space for exoneration: for instance, of anaesthetists who privileged a diagnosis of status lymphaticus over the dangers from the chloroform they administered, of law enforcement officers who have claimed excited delirium as a defence. Too often, certain diagnoses have shown themselves to be a form of obfuscation; a repudiation of the search for answers or accountability. Some of the people we have met in this book were turned into patients when they should not have been. The diagnoses foisted upon them sanctioned, even legitimised, unforgivable treatments – the electric shocks Jeremy was subjected to, or the tranquilisers injected repeatedly into the veins of allegedly psychotic and drug-addled men in Handsworth. Value-laden diagnoses have the potential to deny the vulnerable the care that they deserve, even as they are based on the slimmest evidence – as the families of children diagnosed with oppositional defiant disorder are discovering, and the women whose babies are removed from them moments after delivery, based on (often alleged) alcohol consumption.

So, what is the way forwards? I want to make a case for change, and for how it might begin.

Firstly, we must consider the question of who gets to construct our diagnoses. The influential mainstream journals where articles are published and the conferences where consensus is reached tend to privilege specialist clinicians and researchers. Overwhelmingly, viewpoints are filtered through a western lens. We should ask: how well represented are the family doctors who will likely see the diagnosed through their lifetime medical journey? Even more importantly, do those attendees and authors embody the groups who are most likely to receive such a diagnosis – who, for instance in the cases of cannabis psychosis, schizophrenia or excited delirium, are overwhelmingly from the black community? There is of course a pressing need to address systemic injustices and inequality beyond the level of individual conferences and journals. But as a first step, we can at least pull up more chairs to the table, listen to multiple perspectives and ensure they meaningfully shape the conversation.

Secondly, we should consider how external actors far from the medical front line influence our diagnostic labels, for better or for worse – the media, the pharmaceutical industry, law enforcement, religious organisations and commercial entities. Reporting conflicts of interest becomes crucial. A pathologist who reports excited delirium should be obliged to declare their links to CED manufacturers, for example. The medical establishment should certainly not have a monopoly on the diagnostic system, but we should not allow these non-medical actors to hide in the shadows either. We must at least understand how these institutional structures fit together.

Thirdly, de-diagnosis should be as integral to clinical encounters as diagnosis. When doctors choose a treatment for their patients, such as chemotherapy, they re-evaluate that treatment at the next appointment. Is it effective, is it causing harm, does it need to be modified or even rejected entirely? The same approach should be applied to diagnosis. An annual 'de-diagnosis' or 'diagnosis rethink' appointment could act as a way forwards. On the same note, diagnoses are rarely deleted at consensus conferences – instead, they are refined. But this approach risks further authenticating an already contentious label. When researchers present their findings of a 10% mortality rate in excited delirium, we tend to question whether that rate might become higher or lower, rather than questioning the legitimacy of, or the harm potentially caused by, the diagnosis itself. If there are several conference sessions that allow for refinement of a diagnosis, should there not be at least just one where the very validity and rationality of a diagnosis, and the biases that surround it, are debated? What rights and responsibilities might this diagnosis confer? Not necessarily to debate whether it is 'real' or not, but whether it serves the diagnosed? Sometimes the construct of diagnosis is more damaging than not having a diagnosis at all.

Making space for this kind of debate and testing of definitions and hypotheses should do nothing to detract from the nobility of medicine. I am enormously proud of the work I have been able to do as a doctor over the past fifteen years, much of which is a testament to the power of diagnostic labels that others designed before me and I was able to deliver to my patients. I have not set out to conduct a polemical attack on the diagnostic process, but rather a hopeful acknowledgement that there is room for transformation, perhaps even revolution.

I truly believe that patients and those who support them have the ability to drive that revolution. The stories I have gathered convince me of it: the activists who helped to banish homosexuality as a psychiatric diagnosis; the Vietnam War veterans who successfully fought for the recognition of PTSD; and Tippa Naphtali, who continues to dispel the myths around excited delirium, in memory of his cousin Mikey Powell.

Of all the accounts I have heard in the course of writing this book, one of the most compelling was Jeremy's. After he first spoke to a journalist about his experiences in 2017, the RCPsych issued an apology to him and others who had endured aversion therapy. Its then president, Wendy Burn, expressed 'profound regret' for the lifelong impact of such 'wholly unethical' practices:

> There are no words that can repair the damage done to anyone who has ever been deemed 'mentally unwell' simply for loving a person of the same sex. For those who were then 'treated' using non-evidence based procedures by mental health professionals up until as late as the 1970s, the trauma of such experiences can never be erased [...]. We can't re-write history, but what we can do is make it clear that today our doors are open and that principles of equality and diversity will be passionately upheld.

There is still a long way to go, but the medical establishment has shown a capacity to acknowledge its mistakes and pledge to do better. Repeatedly, many within the establishment have bravely forced change.

The diagnosed have powerfully started these dialogues, valiantly propelled them, and audaciously defined them. I hope that those who have spoken here might inspire us all to bear witness to their struggles, to support them in their journey towards care and compassion, and to try to right the wrongs that we see.

Notes

ix   *'a man without ideas'*. V. Igreja, B. Dias-Lambranca and A. Richters, '*Gamba* spirits, gender relations, and healing in post-civil war Gorongosa, Mozambique', *Journal of the Royal Anthropological Institute*, 14 (2008): 353–71.

xiii   *'very much interrupted'*. J. Parkinson, *An Essay on the Shaking Palsy* (London: Sherwood, Neely and Jones, 1817).

xvi   *'around the world'*. E. Aarseth et al., 'Scholars' open debate paper on the World Health Organization ICD-11 Gaming Disorder proposal', *Journal of Behavioural Addictions*, 6/3 (2017): 267–70.

xvi   *'field of medicine'*. Annemarie Jutel, *Putting a Name to It: Diagnosis in Contemporary Society* (Baltimore, MD: Johns Hopkins University Press, 2011).

xvii   *'rearranging their prejudices'*. This quote has been erroneously attributed to various people, including the philosopher and psychologist William James. In 1906, the *Zion's Herald* reported them as the words of a Bishop Oldham, probably William Fitzjames Oldham (see vol. 84, no. 45, 7 Nov 1906, p. 1433, col. 2).

xviii   *and 'reformist delusions'*. K. W. De Pauw, 'Psychiatry in the Soviet Union', *Nature*, 332/774 (1988): 774.

xx   *'or several locks'*. J. J. Pruszyński, J. Putz and D. Cianciara, 'Plica neuropathica – A short history and description of a

233

particular case', *Hygeia Public Health*, 48 (2013): 481–5.

xx *'a bird's nest'*. V. Ramya Maduri, A. Vedachalam and S. Kiruthika, '"Castor Oil" – the culprit of acute hair felting', *International Journal of Trichology*, 9/3 (2017): 116–18.

xx *to that diagnosis*. E. Sakalauskaitė-Juodeikienė, P. Eling and S. Finger, 'Stephanus Bisius (1724–1790) on mania and melancholy, and the disorder called *plica polonica*', *Journal of the History of the Neurosciences*, 30/1 (2021): 77–93.

xx *'conceive they recover'*. J. Lange, *De morbo virgineo. Epistola XXI, Epistolae Medicinales (1554)*, trans. R. Major, *Classic descriptions of disease*, 2nd edn (Springfield, IL and Baltimore, MD: Charles C. Thomas, 1932).

xxi *the City of London, by 1800*. I. S. Loudon, 'Chlorosis, anaemia, and anorexia nervosa', *BMJ*, 281/6256 (1980): 1669–75.

xxi *'its victim an object as hideous to behold'* . F. Guesnet, 'Body, place, and knowledge: the plica polonica in travelogues and experts' reflections around 1800', *Central Europe*, 17/1 (2019): 54–66.

xxi *'modern corsets'*. Josep Bernabeu-Mestre et al., eds, *La topografía médica d'Ontinyent de 1916* (Ontinyent: Ayuntamiento de Ontinyent, 2004), pp. 191–3.

xxii *in its millions*. See J. Wilcock and D. Taylor 'Polycystic ovarian syndrome: overdiagnosed and overtreated?', *British Journal of General Practice* 68/670 (2018): 243; and T. Copp et al., 'Are expanding disease definitions unnecessarily labelling women with polycystic ovary syndrome?', *BMJ*, 358/8118 (2017).

xxii *'coffee beans'*. K. Figlio, 'Chlorosis and chronic disease in 19th-century Britain: the social constitution of somatic illness in a capitalist society', *International Journal of Health Services*, 8/4 (1978): 589–617.

xxiv *'ganja junkies'*. Philip Lymn, *Evening Mail*, 2 Oct 1985.

xxiv *'Zulu-style war cries'*. Rachel Yemm, 'Immigration, race, and local media in the Midlands: 1960–1985', PhD thesis, University of Lincoln, 2018, p. 261. See also 'US embassy cables: Ambassador labels mid-80s Britain as "Dickensian" after race riots', *Guardian*, 28 Nov 2010.

1   *disciplined themselves to obey them.* (Cambridge, MA: Harvard University Press, 1978), p. 3.

2   *one in five people.* L. Shaw-Taylor, 'An introduction to the history of infectious diseases, epidemics and the early phases of the long-run decline in mortality', *Economic History Review*, 73/3 (2020): E1–19.

2   *in the 1831–2 outbreak.* E. Ashworth Underwood, 'The history of cholera in Great Britain', meeting report, *Journal of the Royal Society of Medicine*, 1 Mar 1948: 165–73.

2   *'great relief from the vapour'.* P. Vinten-Johansen et al., *Cholera, Chloroform, and the Science of Medicine: A Life of John Snow* (Oxford: OUP, 2003), p. 369.

2   *'delightful beyond measure'.* Tony Allen-Mills, '"Blessed chloroform" eased Victoria's eighth labour', *Sunday Times*, 16 Feb 2020.

3   *'from a … reporter'.* B. L. Ligon, 'Louis Pasteur: a controversial figure in a debate on scientific ethics', *Seminars in Pediatric Infectious Diseases*, 13/2 (2002): 134–41.

4   *'problem in medicine'.* A. Dally, 'Status lymphaticus: sudden death in children from "visitation of God" to cot death', *Medical History*, 41/1 (1997): 70–85.

4   *'to which the human frame is subject'.* Albert H. Hayes, *The Science of Life; or, Self-Preservation. A Medical Treatise on Nervous and Physical Disability, Spermatorrhoea, Impotence and Sterility* (Boston, MA: Peabody Medical Institute, 1868), p. 121.

4   *'ravages society'.* D. Hodgson, 'Spermatomania—the English response to Lallemand's disease', *Journal of the Royal Society of Medicine*, 98/8 (2005): 375–9.

5   *'instead of standing'*. Ellen Bayuk Rosenman, *Unauthorized Pleasures* (Ithaca, NY: Cornell University Press, 2018), pp. 16–49.

5   *seventh century AD*. A. Sumathipala, S. H. Siribaddana and D. Bhugra, 'Culture-bound syndromes: the story of dhat syndrome', *British Journal of Psychiatry*, 184/3 (2004): 200–9.

5   *'becoming "womanish"'*. *On the Seed*, as quoted by Peter Brown, *The Body and Society: Men, Women and Sexual Renunciation in Early Christianity* (London: Faber and Faber, 1985), p. 11.

5   *'to their Graves'. Onania, or the Heinous Sin of Self-Pollution, and All Its Frightful Consequences (in Both Sexes) Considered*, 20th edn (Glasgow: A. Mackintosh, *c.*1760), p. 23.

6   *'stunted in growth'*. Richard Dawson, *An Essay on Spermatorrhœa, and Urinary Deposits, With Observations of the Nature, Causes, and Treatment of Various Disorders of the Generative System*, 6th edn (London: Aylott and Jones, 1852).

6   *'with the hand'*. William Acton, *The Functions and Disorders of the Reproductive Organs in Childhood, Youth, Adult Age, and Advanced Life* (London: J. & A. Churchill, 1875), pp. 25, 279.

7   *'the bud of our progress'*. T. Wakley, 'Homeopathic quackery', *Lancet*, 15 May 1858: 483–5.

7   *'obtained by a visit'*. *Lancet*, 'Medical News', 26 Apr 1851: 474.

8   *'rode in the park'*. A. W. Bates, 'Dr Kahn's Museum: obscene anatomy in Victorian London', Journal of the Royal Society of Medicine, 99/12 (2006): 618–24.

8   *a very great extent. Handbook of Dr. Kahn's Museum* (London: W. Snell, 1863), pp. 71–2.

8   *'the leading medical men'*. *Lancet*, 'Medical News', 13 Aug 1853.

9   *'respect public decency'*. 'The action against Kahn, of Coventry Street, for extortion: suppression of obscene quackery', *Lancet*, 15 Aug 1857.

9   *'filthy handbills'*. E. Stephens, 'Pathologizing leaky male

bodies: spermatorrhea in nineteenth-century British medicine and popular anatomical museums', *Journal of the History of Sexuality*, 17/3 (2008): 421–38.

9   *'such as Kahn's'*. Ibid.

9   *and flag officers*. A. W. Bates, '"Indecent and demoralising representations": public anatomy museums in mid-Victorian England', *Medical History*, 52/1 (2008): 1–22.

10   *'any professional respect'*. M. J. D. Roberts, 'The politics of professionalization: MPs, medical men, and the 1858 Medical Act', *Medical History*, 53/1 (2009): 37–56.

10   *'graverobbers'*. T. M. Parssinen, 'Professional deviants and the history of medicine: medical mesmerists in Victorian Britain', *The Sociological Review*, 27/1, supplement (1979): 103–20.

11   *aligned them with tradesmen*. Ellen Bayuk Rosenman, 'Body doubles: the spermatorrhea panic', *Journal of the History of Sexuality*, 12/3 (2003): 365–99.

11   *Quack Prosecution Fund*. Bates, '"Indecent and Demoralising Representations"'.

11   *'back to the defendants'*. Bates, 'Dr Kahn's Museum'.

12   *from the 1850s onwards*. C. Benninghaus, 'Beyond constructivism?: gender, medicine and the early history of sperm analysis, Germany 1870–1900', *Gender and History*, 24 (2012): 647–76.

13   *not be too late*. 'Patient letters to Dr Kahn', in *Handbook of Dr Kahn's Museum*, p. 180.

13   *'there can be no doubt'*. John Laws Milton, 'On the nature and treatment of spermatorrhœa', *Lancet*, 4 March 1854: 243–6.

13   *carried too far*. Robert Bartholow, *Spermatorrhoea: Its Causes, Symptoms, Results and Treatment*, 4th edn, (New York: William Wood and Co., 1879), pp. 78–9, 93–5.

14   *'a theory to prove'*. George G. Gascoyen, 'On spermatorrhoea and its treatment', *BMJ*, 1/577 (1872): 67–9.

14   *'unknown among Englishmen'*. D. Hodgson, 'Spermatomania—
      the English response to Lallemand's disease', *Journal of the
      Royal Society of Medicine*, 98/8 (2005): 375–9.

14   *for several decades*. R. Darby, 'Pathologizing male sexuality:
      Lallemand, spermatorrhea, and the rise of circumcision',
      Journal of the History of Medicine and Allied Sciences, 60/3
      (2005): 283–319.

14   *were now implicated*. James Paget, *Clinical Lectures and Essays*
      (New York: D. Appleton, 1875).

15   *'human vivisection'*. C. Brock, 'Risk, responsibility and surgery
      in the 1890s and early 1900s', *Medical History*, 57/3 (2013):
      317–37.

15   *wills and testaments*. G. C. Alter and A. G. Carmichael
      'Classifying the dead: toward a history of the registration of
      causes of death', *Journal of the History of Medicine and Allied
      Sciences*, 54/2 (1999): 114–32.

16   *'prest and trod to death'*. Craig Spence, *Accidents and Violent
      Death in Early Modern London 1650–1750* (Woodbridge,
      Suffolk: Boydell Press, 2016), p. 25.

16   *'at St Giles Cripplegate'*. 'Bills of Mortality for 21–28 Feb
      1664', in *London's Dreadful Visitation: Or, a Collection of All the
      Bills of Mortality for This Present Year* (London: E. Cotes, 1665).

16   *sometimes illiterate*. R. Munkhoff, 'Poor women and parish
      public health in sixteenth-century London', *Renaissance
      Studies*, 28/4 (2014): 579–96.

16   *30 per week*. Leeds Barroll, *Politics, Plague, and Shakespeare's
      Theater: The Stuart Years* (Cornell University Press, Ithaca,
      1991).

17   *was facing growing criticism as a result*. Edward Higgs, *Life,
      Death and Statistics: Civil Registration, Censuses and the Work
      of the General Register Office, 1836–1952* (Hatfield: Local
      Population Studies, 2004).

17   *provided specific forms.* A. Hardy. '"Death is the cure of all diseases": using the General Register Office cause of death statistics for 1837–1920', *Social History of Medicine*, 7/3 (1994): 472–92.

18   *'who give certificates'.* Supplement to the Thirty-Fifth Annual Report of the Registrar General of Births, Marriades and Deaths (London: HMSO, 1875), p. lxxx.

18   *incompetence or worse.* A. Hardy, '"Death is the cure of all diseases"'.

18   *and poor sanitation.* G. H. H. Glasgow, 'The campaign for medical coroners in nineteenth-century England and its aftermath: a Lancashire focus on failure (Part I)', *Mortality*, 9/2 (2004): 150–67.

19   *'the fees of the coroner'.* Hansard, HC Deb 28 May 1851 vol 117 cc100–13.

19   *'a discrete entity'.* D. Armstrong, 'The invention of infant mortality', *Sociology of Health & Illness*, 8/3 (1986): 211–32.

19   *'takes away life'.* 'University College and St. Bartholomew's Hospitals: Deaths from Inhalation of Chloroform', *Lancet*, 29 Oct 1853.

19   *'for general use'.* 'Chloroform Accidents', *BMJ*, 2/465 (1869): 589–91.

20   *died suddenly while swimming.* A. Paltauf, 'Über die Beziehungen des Thymus zum plötzlichen Tod' ('Associations between the thymus and sudden death'), *Wiener klinische Wochenschrift*, 46 (1889): 877–81.

20   *'the present report'.* BMA, 'Final report of special chloroform committee', *BMJ*, 2/2584 (1910): 47–72.

20   *operation or not.* A. Dally, 'Status lymphaticus'.

20   *thought to be present.* 'The annus medicus', *Lancet*, ii, 25 Dec 1909: 1899–900.

21   *'short-necked'.* J. F. Taylor, 'Status lymphaticus', *Proceedings of*

the Royal Society of Medicine, 33 (1939): 119–25.

21   *were supportive*. D. Symmers, 'The cause of sudden death in status lymphaticus', *American Journal of Diseases of Children*, 14/6 (1917): 463–9.

21   *'that the infant's father provided'*. A. E. Oestreich, 'William H. Crane of Cincinnati and the first irradiation of the pediatric thymus, 1905', *American Journal of Roentgenology*, 165/5 (1995): 1064–5.

22   *in early life*. B. J. Duffy Jr. and P. J. Fitzgerald, 'Thyroid cancer in childhood and adolescence; a report on 28 cases', *Cancer*, 3/6 (1950): 1018–32.

22   *'the administration of an anaesthetic'*. *Seventy-Fourth Annual Report of the Registrar General of Births, Deaths and Marriages* (London: HMSO, 1911), p. xcii.

22   *registrars or coroners*. *Lancet*, 1 October 1910: 1020–3.

23   *'medical mythology'*. Major Greenwood and Hilda M. Woods, '"Status Thymico-Lymphaticus" considered in the light of Recent Work on the Thymus', *Journal of Hygiene*, 26/3 (1927): 305–26.

23   *longer than it should*. 'The end of status lymphaticus', *Lancet*, 14 Mar 1931: 593–4.

23   *until 1940*. D. J. Steward, 'Sudden unexpected death during pediatric anesthesia: from status thymico–lymphaticus to silent cardiomyopathy', *Paediatric Anaesthesia*, 23/11 (2013): 1101–3.

25   *and sexual impotence*. George Miller Beard, *American nervousness: Its causes and consequences* (New York: G. P. Putnam's Sons, 1881).

25   *'whose powers of resistance are weakest'*. J. S. Greene, 'Neurasthenia; its causes and its treatment', *Boston Medical and Surgical Journal*, 109/4 (1883): 75–8.

25   *'trifling with Mrs. D.'*. *Theodore Dreiser: American Diaries 1902–*

1926, ed. Thomas P. Riggio (Philadelphia: University of Pennsylvania Press, 1983), p. 77.

25 *'darkness of neurasthenia'*. *A Backward Glance*, in *Novellas and Other Writings* (New York: The Library of America, 1990), p. 1025.

26 *metropolitan cities*. C. Hirschman and E. Mogford, 'Immigration and the American industrial revolution from 1880 to 1920', *Social Science Research*, 38/4 (2009): 897–920.

26 *'the present day'*. E. H. van Deusen, 'Observations on a form of nervous prostration (neurasthenia) culminating in insanity', *American Journal of Insanity*, 25/4 (1869): 445–61.

26 *'mental repose'*. *On Mental Strain and Overwork* (Lewes: G. P. Barton, 1875), p. 11.

26 *'if not injurious'*. Beard, *American Nervousness*.

26 *330 patients*. J. Collins and C. Phillips, 'The etiology and treatment of neurasthenia: An analysis of three hundred and thirty-three cases', *Medical Record*, 55 (1899): 413–21.

27 *'distinguished malady'*. Beard, *American Nervousness*.

27 *'as long as you live'*. *The Living of Charlotte Perkins Gilman: An Autobiography* (Madison, WI: University of Winsconsin Press, 1990), p. 96.

27 *places of amusement*. W. B. Stewart, 'Neurasthenia and Its Treatment', *JAMA*, 32/8 (1899): 438.

28 *clinics in Germany*. D. Kaufmann, 'Neurasthenia in Wilhelmine Germany: culture, sexuality, and the demands of nature', *Clio Medica*, 63 (2001): 161–76.

28 *'hardly another pathological phenomenon'*. 'Nervosität und neurasthenische Zustände' ('Nervousness and neurasthenic states'), in Hermann Nothnagel, ed., *Specielle Pathologie und Therapie* ('Special pathology and therapy') (Vienna: Alfred Holder, 1899), p. 50.

28 *'function of the nervous system'*. 'Neurasthenia: the wear

and tear of life', *BMJ*, 1903/1 (1903): 1017.

28   *corsets and bustles.* L. Goering, '"Russian nervousness": neurasthenia and national identity in nineteenth-century Russia', *Medical History*, 47/1 (2003): 23–46.

28   *'incoherent symptoms'.* C. Sengoopta, '"A mob of incoherent symptoms"? Neurasthenia in British medical discourse, 1860–1920', in Marijke Gijswijt-Hofstra and Roy Porter, eds, *Cultures of Neurasthenia from Beard to the First World War* (New York: Rodopi, 2001), pp. 97–115.

29   *brain tumour diagnoses.* R. E. Taylor, 'Death of neurasthenia and its psychological reincarnation: a study of neurasthenia at the National Hospital for the Relief and Cure of the Paralysed and Epileptic, Queen Square, London, 1870–1932', *British Journal of Psychiatry*, 179 (2001): 550–7.

29   *had the condition.* Thomas D. Savill, *Clinical lectures on Neurasthenia* (London: Glaisher, 1899).

29   *'incapacitating conditions'.* 'Hysteria and Neurasthenia', *Brain*, 27/1 (1904): 1–26.

29   *'American civilization'.* Beard, *American Nervousness*.

29   *'disease of America'.* E. Wakefield, 'Nervousness: the national disease of America', *McClure's Magazine*, 2 (1894): 302–7.

29   *'in-door classes'.* Beard, *American Nervousness*, p. 26.

29   *'possessed such maladies'.* Ibid., pp. 7–8.

30   *'chiselled features'.* Ibid., p. 26.

30   *'human capacity'.* J. S. Greene, *Neurasthenia: Its Causes and Its Home Treatment* (Cambridge, MA: Riverside Press, 1883), p. 5.

30   *'the plane of a superior'.* 'Neurasthenia: the traumatic neuroses and psychoses', in William Osler and Thomas McCrae, eds, *Modern Medicine: Its Theory and Practice* (Philadelphia: Lea & Febiger, 1910).

30   *the non-tropical form.* A. Crozier, 'What was tropical about

tropical neurasthenia? The utility of the diagnosis in the management of British East Africa', *Journal of the History of Medicine and Allied Sciences*, 64/4 (2009): 518–48.

31 *in government service at home.* H. C. Squires, quoted by an anonymous BMA member in 'Tropical Neurasthenia', *East African Medical Journal*, 'Correspondence', 12 (1935–6): 28.

31 *otherwise fairly fit.* R. Havelock Charles, 'Neurasthenia, and its bearing on the decay of Northern peoples in India', *Transactions of The Royal Society of Tropical Medicine and Hygiene*, 7/1 (1913): 2–31.

31 *'or using them'.* Ibid.

32 *'as one has seen'.* R. van Someren, 'Mental irritability and breakdown in the tropics', *BMJ*, 1/3404 (1926): 596.

32 *'criminal folly'.* M. McKinnon, 'Medical aspects of white settlement in Kenya', *East African Medical Journal*, 11 (1934–5): 389.

33 *'neurasthenic symptoms'.* Cited in Aldo Castellani, *Climate and Acclimatization: Some Notes and Observations* (London: John Bale, Sons & Danielsson, 1931), 53–5.

33 *'in the British Civil Service'.* Francis George Heath, *The British Civil Service: Home, Colonial, Indian and Diplomatic* (London: Grafton & Co., 1915).

33 *'climatic influences'.* Havelock Charles, 'Neurasthenia'.

33 *'characterize them all'.* S. E. Jelliffe, 'Dispensary work in nervous diseases', *Journal of Nervous and Mental Disease*, 32 (1905): 449–53.

34 *'American civilization'.* Robert Carroll, *The Mastery of Nervousness Based Upon Self Reeducation* (New York: The MacMillan Company, 1917).

34 *'the higher race'.* Francis Galton, *Inquiries into Human Faculty and its Development* (London: Macmillan & Co., 1883), 25–7.

34   *'segregated in early life'*. Frederick Mott, 'Is insanity on the increase?', *Sociological Review*, 6 (1913): 1–29.

34   *'future generations'*. 'Leading Churchill Myths', International Churchill Society, 17 Apr 2013, https://winstonchurchill. org/publications/finest-hour/finest-hour-152/leading-churchill-myths-churchills-campaign-against-the-feeble-minded-was-deliberately-omitted-by-his-biographers/.

34   *'certainly be killed'*. Anne Olivier Bell and Andrew McNellie, eds, *The Diary of Virginia Woolf*, Vol. 1 (San Diego: Harcourt Brace and Company, 1977), p. 13.

34   *'inferior infants'*. Marie Carmichael Stopes, *Radiant Motherhood: A Book for Those Who are Creating the Future* (London: G. P. Putnam's Sons, 1920).

35   *of the Reich*. Letter to Von Strümpell, 2 Feb 1919, quoted in Jürgen Pfeiffer, *Hirnforschung in Deutschland 1849 bis 1974* ('Brain research in Germany 1849–1974'), trans. author (Berlin: Springer, 2004), p. 400.

35   *forced sterilisation*. A. Karenberg et al., 'Historical review: a short history of German neurology – from its origins to the 1940s', *Neurological Research and Practice*, 1/14 (2019).

35   *disappeared entirely after 1941*. R. E. Taylor, 'Death of neurasthenia'.

36   *'and the nation'*. Tsung-yi Lin, 'Neurasthenia revisited: its place in modern psychiatry', *Culture, Medicine, and Psychiatry*, 13/2 (1989): 105–29.

36   *'sexual immorality'*. S. Frühstück, 'Male anxieties: nerve force, nation, and the power of sexual knowledge', *Journal of the Royal Asiatic Society*, 15/1 (2005): 71–88.

36   *and their families*. P. McDonald-Scott, S. Machizawa and H. Satoh, 'Diagnostic disclosure: a tale in two cultures', *Psychological Medicine*, 22/1 (1992): 147–57.

36   *synonymous with neurasthenia*. A. Farmer et al., 'Neuraesthenia

revisited: ICD-10 and DSM-III-R psychiatric syndromes in chronic fatigue patients and comparison subjects', *British Journal of Psychiatry*, 167/4 (1995): 503–6.

37 *to be the case with neurasthenia*. D. R. Lipsitt, 'Is today's 21st century burnout 19th century's neurasthenia?', *Journal of Nervous and Mental Disease*, 207/9 (2019): 773–7.

43 *'abnormal circumstances'*. WHO, *The ICD-9 Classification of Mental and Behavioural Disorders: Clinical Descriptions and Diagnostic Guide-Lines* (WHO, 1975).

44 *alcoholism and homosexuality*. J. Drescher, 'Out of DSM: depathologizing homosexuality', *Behavioural Sciences*, 5/4 (2015): 565–75.

44 *'who respond to it'*. *Outsiders: Studies in the Sociology of Deviance* (New York: Free Press, 1963), p. 14.

44 *'most brutal persecutions'*. K. M. Benkert, 'An open letter to the Prussian Minister of Justice', trans. M. Lombardi-Nash, in M. Blasius and S. Phelan, eds, *We Are Everywhere: A Historical Sourcebook of Gay and Lesbian Politics* (New York: Routledge, 1997), pp. 67–79.

45 *'is ascendant'*. Eliot Freidson, *Profession of Medicine: A Study of the Sociology of Applied Medicine* (Chicago: University of Chicago Press, 1972), p. 244.

45 *'sociopathic personality disturbances'*. APA, *Diagnostic and Statistical Manual of Mental Disorders* (Washington, DC: APA, 1952).

45 *fabric of the nation*. Supplement 2656, *BMJ* (1955): 2: S165.

46 *'with homosexuality'*. Ibid.

47 *'such institutions'*. Ibid.

47 *'well-being of the community'*. *BMJ*, 'Correspondence', 21 Jan 1956: 171.

47 *'which concerns our own'*. *BMJ*, 'Correspondence', 31 Dec 1955: 1623.

48   *thinly veiled.* Supplement 2656, *BMJ*.

48   *'treatment of homosexuals'*. B. James, 'Case of homosexuality treated by aversion therapy', *BMJ*, 1/5280 (1962): 768–70.

48   *'in other respects'*. *Report of the Committee on Homosexual Offences and Prostitution* (London: HMSO, 1957).

49   *'to Christians'*. Zoë Pollock, 'Psychiatry off a Cliff', *Atlantic*, 30 Dec 2010.

49   *the latter group.* Ernst Pfeiffer, 'Ein geheilter Fall von Homosexualität durch Hodentransplantation' ('Successful use of testicle transplant in curing homosexuality: a case report'), *Deutsche medizinsche Wochenschrift*, 20 (1922): 660–2.

50   *1933 Law Against Habitual Criminals and Sex Offenders.* G. J. Giles, '"The most unkindest cut of all": castration, homosexuality and Nazi justice', *Journal of Contemporary History*, 27/1 (1992): 41–61.

50   *over the same period.* G. Lewis, 'Lifting the ban on gays in the civil service: federal policy toward gay and lesbian employees since the Cold War', *Public Administration Review*, 57/5 (1997): 387–95.

50   *'easy prey to the blackmailer'*. United States Senate, *Employment of Homosexuals and Other Sex Perverts in Government, Interim Report* (Washington, DC: Government Printing Office, 1950).

51   *on the grounds of homosexuality.* United States Supreme Court (ruling), Clive Michael Boutilier v. Immigration and Naturalization Service, 22 Mar 1967, https://www.law. cornell.edu/supremecourt/text/387/118.

51   *'their sound reformation'*. Supplement 2656, *BMJ*.

52   *'I'm going to let them'*. Luchia Fitzgerald, quoted in Alkarim Jivani, *It's Not Unusual: A History of Lesbian and Gay Britain in the Twentieth Century* (London: Michael O'Mara, 1997), pp. 126–27.

53   *'exclusively homosexual'*. K. Freund, 'Some problems in the

treatment of homosexuality', in H. J. Eysenck, ed., *Behaviour Therapy and the Neuroses: Readings in Modern Methods of Treatment Derived From Learning Theory* (London: Pergamon, 1960), pp. 312–26.

53 *and Jean Piaget.* Steven J. Haggblom et al., 'The 100 most eminent psychologists of the 20th century', *Review of General Psychology*, 6/2 (2002): 139–52.

54 *agreed with their judgments.* Claire Hilton and Tom Stephenson, eds, *Psychiatric Hospitals in the UK in the 1960s (Witness Seminar), 11 Oct 2019* (London: RCPsych, 2020), p. 34.

54 *studies were 'unsafe'.* Hans Eysenck and Ronald Grossarth-Maticek, 'King's College London enquiry into publications', May 2019, https://www.kcl.ac.uk/news/statements/docs/hans-eysenck-enquiry-final-may-2019.pdf.

54 *'a full-length novel'.* B. James, 'Case of homosexuality treated by aversion therapy'.

55 *'in this country'.* S. Howard 'Aversion therapy for homosexuality', *BMJ*, 1/5286 (1962): 1206–7.

55 *'establish its value'.* *BMJ*, 'Correspondence', 21 Apr 1962.

55 *'can be cured'.* *Observer*, 18 Mar 1962; *Sunday Pictorial*, 5 Feb 1961.

55 *only decades later.* 'Gay injustice was "widespread"', BBC News, 12 Sep 2009, news.bbc.co.uk/1/hi/uk/8251033.stm.

55 *wrote in 1970.* M. MacCulloch and M. Feldman, 'Aversion therapy of homosexuality', *British Journal of Psychiatry*, 116/535 (1970): 673–6.

56 *Lancashire and Belfast.* K. Davison, 'Cold War Pavlov: homosexual aversion therapy in the 1960s', *History of the Human Sciences*, 34/1 (2021): 89–119.

56 *treatment unit for homosexuality.* Tommy Dickinson, 'Mental nursing and "sexual deviation": exploring the role of nurses and the experience of former patients, 1935–1974',

PhD thesis, University of Manchester, 2012.

56   *'homosexual direction'*. N. McConaghy, 'Subjective and penile plethysmograph responses following aversion-relief and apomorphine aversion therapy for homosexual impulses', *British Journal of Psychiatry*, 115/523 (1969): 723–30.

57   *rejecting relationships entirely*. J. Bancroft, 'Aversion therapy of homosexuality. A pilot study of 10 cases', *British Journal of Psychiatry*, 115/529 (1969): 1417–31.

57   *sexual deviancy*. I. Rieber and V. Sigusch, 'Psychosurgery on sex offenders and sexual "deviants" in West Germany', *Archives of Sexual Behaviour*, 8/6 (1979): 523–7.

58   *'this problem in man'*. F. Roeder and D. Müller, 'Zur stereotaktischen Heilung der pädophilen Homosexualität' ('The stereotaxic treatment of pedophilic homosexuality'), *Deutsche medizinische Wochenschrift*, 9 (1969): 409–15.

58   *'verbal aggression'*. Ibid.

59   *'the Catholic religion'*. Jeremy Gavins, *"Is It about That Boy?": The Shocking Trauma of Aversion Therapy: A Memoir* ([n. pl.]: JGSCR Publishing, 2018).

60   *'a patient demands'*. Tommy Dickinson, *'Mental nursing'*.

60   *homosexual patients*. M. King, G. Smith and A. Bartlett, 'Treatments of homosexuality in Britain since the 1950s – an oral history: the experience of professionals', *BMJ*, 328/7437 (2004): 429.

61   *one way or the other*. Claudia Dreifus, *'A conversation with John Bancroft – sitting in the ultimate hot seat: the Kinsey Institute'*, *The New York Times*, 25 May 1999.

62   *'poison in my mind'*. Beverly D'Silva, 'When gay meant mad', *Independent*, 3 Aug 1996.

62   *'"cure" homosexuality'*. J. Drescher, 'Out of DSM'.

63   *'your sickness talking'*. B. Gittings, 'Show and tell', *Journal of Gay & Lesbian Mental Health*, 12/3 (2008): 289–95.

63   *'our social mores'*. J. Marmor, 'A symposium: should homo-
     sexuality be in the APA nomenclature?', *American Journal of
     Psychiatry*, 130/11 (1973): 1207–16.

64   *his own profession*. B. Gittings, 'Show and tell'.

64   *'our dooms sealed'*. D. L. Scasta, 'John E. Fryer, MD, and the
     Dr. H. Anonymous episode', *Journal of Gay and Lesbian
     Psychotherapy*, 6/4 (2003): 73–84.

64   *'what they saw!'*. B. Gittings, 'Show and tell'.

64   *psychological maladjustment*. E. Hooker, 'The adjustment of the
     male overt homosexual', *Journal of Projective Techniques*, 21/1
     (1957): 18–31.

65   *rationalisation for discrimination*. J. Drescher, 'The removal of
     homosexuality from the DSM: its impact on today's marriage
     equality debate', *Journal of Gay & Lesbian Mental Health*, 16/2
     (2012): 124–135.

65   *'Hampstead and Highgate'*. M. L. Ellis, 'Lesbians, gay men
     and psychoanalytic training', *Free Associations*, 4/32 (1994):
     501–17.

66   *'And I still do'*. M. King et al., 'Treatments of homosexuality
     in Britain'.

66   *'the bringing up of children'*. Supplement 2656, *BMJ*, *op. cit.*

66   *same-sex relationships*. S. Carr and H. Spandler, 'Hidden
     from history? A brief modern history of the psychiatric
     "treatment" of lesbian and bisexual women in England',
     Lancet Psychiatry, 6/4 (2019): 289–90.

69   *'religious freedom'*. 'Government sets out plan to ban
     conversion therapy', 11 May 2021, https://www.gov.uk/
     government/news/government-sets-out-plan-to-ban-
     conversion-therapy.

70   *should be legal*. Ipsos, 'Ipsos Poll Conducted for Reuters:
     Stonewall Anniversary Poll 06.06.2019', https://www.ipsos.
     com/sites/default/files/ct/news/documents/2019-06/

2019_reuters_tracking_-_stonewall_anniversary_
poll_06_07_2019.pdf.

70   *'or spiritual advisors'*. C. Mallory, T. N. T. Brown and K. J.
Conron, 'Conversion therapy and LGBT youth: update',
UCLA School of Law, Williams Institute, Jun 2019, https://
williamsinstitute.law.ucla.edu/wp-content/uploads/
Conversion-Therapy-Update-Jun-2019.pdf.

70   *internalised homophobia*. UNHCR, *Report on Conversion Therapy*,
May 2020, https://www.ohchr.org/EN/Issues/SexualOrien
tationGender/Pages/ReportOnConversiontherapy.aspx.

70   *'potentially harmful'*. Church of England, 'General Synod
backs ban on conversion therapy', 8 Jul 2017, https://
www.churchofengland.org/news-and-media/news-and-
statements/general-synod-backs-ban-conversion-therapy.

71   *on London buses*. R. Clucas, 'Sexual orientation change efforts,
conservative Christianity and resistance to sexual justice',
Social Sciences, 6/54 (2017): 1–49.

71   *'Jesus Christ'*. Core Issues Trust (statement), 'Truth is stranger
than it used to be: when "puffing" isn't lying', 11 Jun 2015,
https://www.core-issues.org/UserFiles/File/Statements/
Statements_2015/CIT_Statement_11_June_2015_Truth_
is_Stranger_than_it_used_to_be_when_puffing_isn_t_
lying.pdf).

71   *'mind of Christ'*. Dr Carys Moseley, 'Why Christians must
defeat the global attack on "conversion therapy" for
homosexuality', Christian Concern, 10 Dec 2018, https://
christianconcern.com/comment/why-christians-must-
defeat-the-global-attack-on-conversion-therapy-for-
homosexuality.

71   *House of Lords peers*. Adam Bychawski, 'UK Christian
"reactionaries" mark 10 years of lobbying against women's
and LGBT rights', Open Democracy, 25 Oct 2018, https://

www.opendemocracy.net/en/5050/christian-concern-reactionaries-10-years-lobbying-women-and-lgbt-rights/.

71   *'masturbation and prostitution'*. 'The *Evening Standard* published an advert from a "pray the gay away" church', BuzzFeed, 26 May 2017, https://www.buzzfeed.com/marieleconte/the-evening-standard-published-an-advert-from-a-pray-the.

72   *'harm to many people'*. Jonathan Merritt, 'The downfall of the ex-gay movement', *Atlantic*, 6 Oct 2015.

78   *vehicles were damaged*. J. Silverman, *Report of an Independent Inquiry into the Handsworth Disturbances* (Birmingham: City of Birmingham, 1985), p. 54.

79   *'sub-post office'*. Les Back and John Solomos, *Race, Politics and Social Change* (London: Routledge, 2002), p. 82.

79   *'Whites and Asians'*. J. Silverman, *Report of an Independent Inquiry*.

80   *'encouraged the mob'*. Jo Thomas, 'New riots erupt in an English city; official attacked', *The New York Times*, 11 Sep 1985.

80   *against black applicants*. C. Brown and the Policy Studies Institute, *Black and White Britain: The Third PSI Survey* (London: Heineman Educational, 1984).

81   *arrestable offence*. Joseph Maggs, 'Fighting Sus! Then and now', Institute of Race Relations, 4 Apr 2019 https://irr.org.uk/article/fighting-sus-then-and-now.

81   *'cause of the riots'*. J. Silverman, *Report of an Independent Inquiry*.

82   *psychosis and violence*. See Philip Lymn, *Evening Mail*, 2 Oct 1985.

82   *'bursting at the seams'*. Ibid.

82   *'mad on drugs'*. Jo Thomas, 'New riots erupt'.

82   *'majoon shop'*. James H. Mills, *Cannabis Britannica: Empire, Trade, and Prohibition, 1800–1928* (Oxford: OUP, 2003).

83   *'do cause insanity'*. W. Mackworth Young, *Report of the Indian*

Hemp Drugs Commission, 1893–94 (Simpla: Office of the Superintendent of Government Printing, 1895).

83   *weak-minded.* G. F. W. Ewens, 'Insanity following the use of indian hemp', *Indian Medical Gazette*, 39/11 (1904): 401–13.

84   *'time in Morocco'.* J. C. Nigrete, 'Psychological adverse effects of cannabis smoking: a tentative classification', *Canadian Medical Association Journal*, 108/2 (1973): 195–202.

84   *only around 60%.* R. Littlewood, 'Community-initiated research: a study of psychiatrists' conceptualisations of "cannabis psychosis"', *Psychiatric Bulletin*, 12/1 (1988): 486–8.

85   *either causes the other.* Carl L. Hart and Charles Ksir, 'Does marijuana use really cause psychotic disorders?', *Observer*, 20 Jan 2019.

85   *and sex education.* H. Altman and R. C. Evenson, 'Marijuana use and subsequent psychiatric symptoms: a replication', *Comprehensive Psychiatry*, 14/5 (1973): 415–20.

85   *cannabis use.* S. H. Gage. 'Cannabis and psychosis: triangulating the evidence', *Lancet Psychiatry*, 6/5 (2019): 364–5.

86   *'entertainers, and others'.* R. J. Gerber, *Legalizing Marijuana: Drug Policy Reform and Prohibition Politics* (Westport, CT: Greenwood Press, 2004).

86   *the greatest social menace.* Cited in M. Booth, *Cannabis: A History* (New York: Picador, 2005).

87   *tested for the drug.* R. Littlewood and M. Lipsedge M., *Aliens and Alienists: Ethnic Minorities and Psychiatry* (London: Routledge, 1997).

87   *'(West Indians)'.* R. Littlewood, 'Community-initiated research'.

88   *were African-Caribbean.* C. Ranger, 'Race, culture and "cannabis psychosis": the role of social factors in the construction of a disease category', *Journal of Ethnic and Migration Studies*, 15/3 (1989): 357–69.

88   *and schizophrenia.* D. McGovern and R. V. Cope, 'First psychiatric admission rates of first and second generation Afro Caribbeans', *Social Psychiatry and Psychiatric Epidemiology*, 22/3 (1987): 139–49.

89   *described the riots as 'tribal'.* Rachel Yemm, 'Immigration, race, and local media', p. 261.

89   *Mayhem Mile.* Paul Gilroy, *There Ain't No Black in the Union Jack* (London: Routledge, 2003), p. 238.

90   *multi-racial riot.* J. Silverman, *Report of an Independent Inquiry.*

90   *'unruly soccer fans'.* Jo Thomas, 'Getting at the causes of Britain's latest black eye', *The New York Times*, 15 Sep 1985.

90   *was white.* Michael Keith, *Race, Riots and Policing: Lore and Disorder in a Multi-Racist Society* (London: UCL Press, 1993).

90   *60% were white.* Deborah Platts-Fowler, '"Beyond the riots" – policing in partnership to prevent and contain urban unrest', PhD thesis, University of Leeds, 2016.

90   *'a large minority of Whites'.* D. Thompson, 'Moss Side riots: the night years of anger exploded in an orgy of violence', *Manchester Evening News*, 4 Jul 2011.

90   *'symbol of their oppression'.* T. Bunyan, 'The police against the people', *Race & Class*, 23/2–3 (1981): 153–170.

91   *'pleasing astonishment'.* 'Christmas at the asylum', The Iron Room, 12 Dec 2016, https://theironroom.wordpress.com/2016/12/12/christmas-at-the-asylum/#_ftn2.

92   *between 1975 and 1982.* D. McGovern and R.V. Cope, 'The compulsory detention of males of different ethnic groups, with special reference to offender patients', *British Journal of Psychiatry*, 150/4 (1987): 505–12.

93   *appropriate treatment.* R. Littlewood, 'Community-initiated research'.

93   *often repeatedly so.* G. Glover and G. Malcolm, 'The prevalence of depot neuroleptic treatment among West Indians and

Asians in the London borough of Newham', *Social Psychiatry and Psychiatric Epidemiology*, 23 (1988): 281–4.

94   *long-term toxicity.* E. Y. Chen, G. Harrison and P. J. Standen, 'Management of first episode psychotic illness in Afro-Caribbean patients', *British Journal of Psychiatry*, 158 (1991): 517–22.

95   *'We're coming down hard on soft minds'.* Daniel Bear, 'Adapting, acting out, or standing firm: understanding the place of drugs in the policing of a London borough', PhD thesis, LSE, 2013.

96   *over the same period.* J. B. Kirkbride et al., 'Incidence of schizophrenia and other psychoses in England, 1950–2009: a systematic review and meta-analyses', *PLOS ONE*, 7/3 (2012): e31660.

97   *over 20 years.* M. S. K. Starzer, M. Nordentoft and C. Hjorthøj, 'Rates and predictors of conversion to schizophrenia or bipolar disorder following substance-induced psychosis', *American Journal of Psychiatry*, 175/4 (2018): 343–50.

97   *synonymous with 'white'.* R. Littlewood and M. Lipsedge, 'Psychiatric illness among British Afro-Caribbeans', *BMJ*, 296/6627 (1988): 359.

97   *'emotional disharmony'.* A. Marsden and J. Adams, 'Are you likely to be a happily married woman?', *Ladies Home Journal*, 31 Mar 1949.

98   *'split personality'.* J. M. Metzl, *The protest psychosis: how Schizophrenia became a Black disease* (Boston, MA: Beacon Press, 2010).

99   *'religion and culture'.* W. Bromberg and F. Simon, 'The "protest" psychosis: a special type of reactive psychosis', *Archives of General Psychiatry*, 19/2 (1968): 155–60.

99   *'schizophrenic, armed, and dangerous'.* J. M. Metzl and K. T. MacLeish, 'Mental illness, mass shootings, and the politics of

American firearms', *American journal of public health*, 105/2 (2015): 240–9.

99   *'violent assaults'*. 'FBI adds Negro mental patient to "10 most wanted" list', *Chicago Tribune*, 6 Jul 1966.

100   *'consistent with his delusions'*. *DSM*, 2nd edn (Washington, DC: APA, 1968).

100   *artefacts and masks*. J. M. Metzl, 'Mainstream anxieties about race in antipsychotic drug ads', *Virtual Mentor*, 14/6 (2012): 494–502.

101   *bipolar disorder*. J. M. Metzl, 'Structural health and the politics of African American masculinity', *American Journal of Men's Health*, 7/4, supplement (2013): 68S–72S.

101   *age and social class*. R. Littlewood et al., 'Psychiatric illness among British Afro-Caribbeans': 950.

101   *their parents' generation*. D. McGovern and R. V. Cope, 'First psychiatric admission rates'.

101   *English patient*. K. Halvorsrud et al., 'Ethnic inequalities in the incidence of diagnosis of severe mental illness in England: a systematic review and new meta-analyses for non-affective and affective psychoses', *Social Psychiatry and Psychiatric Epidemiology*, 54 (2019): 1311–23.

101   *there is none*. Jamie D. Brooks and Meredith L. King, *Geneticizing Disease: Implications for Racial Health Disparities* (Washington, DC: Center for American Progress, 2008).

102   *mental health issues*. J. Y. Nazroo, K. S. Bhui and J. Rhodes, 'Where next for understanding race/ethnic inequalities in severe mental illness? Structural, interpersonal and institutional racism', *Sociology of Health and Illness*, 42 (2020): 262–76.

102   *ultimately failed him*. H. Prins, *Report of the Committee of Inquiry into the Death of Orville Blackwood and a Review of the Deaths of Two Other African-Caribbean Patients* (London: SHSA, 1994).

103   *most of them compulsory.* I. Cummins, 'Discussing race, racism and mental health: two mental health inquiries reconsidered', *International Journal of Human Rights in Healthcare*, 8/3 (2015): 160–72.

103   *'stopped breathing'.* 'Inquiry says depot injections can kill', *BMJ*, 'News', 307 (1993): 641.

103   *'attention to duty'.* 'Broadmoor death was accidental: second inquest confirms verdict on patient forcibly injected with drugs', *Independent*, 2 Apr 1993.

104   *restrictive measures.* P. Noble and S. Rodger, 'Violence by psychiatric in-patients', *British Journal of Psychiatry*, 155 (1989): 384–90.

105   *have been detained.* R. Corrigall and D. Bhugra, 'The role of ethnicity and diagnosis in rates of adolescent psychiatric admission and compulsory detention: a longitudinal case-note study', *Journal of the Royal Society of Medicine*, 106/5 (2013): 190–5.

105   *south Asian patients.* P. Barnett et al., 'Ethnic variations in compulsory detention under the Mental Health Act: a systematic review and meta-analysis of international data', *Lancet Psychiatry*, 6/4 (2019): 305–17.

105   *in primary care.* K. Halvorsrud et al., 'Ethnic inequalities and pathways to care in psychosis in England: a systematic review and meta-analysis', *BMC Medicine*, 16/223 (2018).

106   *'has tied the animal'.* J. Ridley and S. Leitch, *Restraint Reduction Network (RRN) Training Standards 2019* (Edgbaston: BILD Publications, 2019).

106   *charges could be brought.* Damien Gayle and Vikram Dodd, 'Mother of man who died after police restraint calls for prosecution', *Guardian*, 9 May 2017.

106   *'couldn't be controlled'.* 'Written evidence from INQUEST (RHR0024)', 22 Sep 2020, https://committees.

parliament.uk/writtenevidence/12268/html.

107 *mental health services.* NICE, *Antisocial Behaviour and Conduct Disorders in Children and Young People: Recognition and Management* (London: NICE, 2017).

107 *at some point in childhood.* APA, 'Diagnostic criteria 313.81 (F91.3)', in *Diagnostic and Statistical Manual of Mental Disorders*, fifth edn (Washington, DC: APA, 2013).

108 *the medical records of community diagnosticians.* K. L. Ballentine, 'Understanding racial differences in diagnosing ODD versus ADHD using critical race theory', *Families in Society*, 100/3 (2019): 282–292.

108 *'reduce yelling and arguing'.* See https://www.semel.ucla.edu/socialskills/research/parenting-children-2-12-years.

109 *family origin.* NICE, *Antisocial behaviour.*

109 *as young as five.* A. R. Todd, K. C. Thiem and R. Neel, 'Does seeing faces of young black boys facilitate the identification of threatening stimuli?', *Psychological Science*, 27/3 (2016): 384–93.

110 *afforded to them.* P. A. Goff et al., 'The essence of innocence: consequences of dehumanizing black children', *Journal of Personality and Social Psychology*, 106/4 (2014): 526–45.

110 *'protect white boys only'.* Vanessa Williams, 'Innocence erased: how society keeps black boys from being boys', 21 Sep 2018.

110 *'19 or 20 years old'.* Ibid.

110 *'lower doses'.* S. H. Meghani, E. Byun and R. M. Gallagher, 'Time to take stock: a meta-analysis and systematic review of analgesic treatment disparities for pain in the United States', *Pain Medicine*, 13 (2012): 150–74.

110 *and appendicitis.* M. Goyal et al., 'Racial disparities in pain management of children with appendicitis in emergency departments', *JAMA Pediatrics*, 169/11 (2015): 996–1002.

111 *chest X-ray.* L. E. Pezzin, P.M. Keyl and G.B. Green, 'Disparities

in the emergency department evaluation of chest pain patients', *Academic Emergency Medicine*, 14 (2007): 149–56.

111   *treat black people's pain adequately.* K. M. Hoffman et al., 'Racial bias in pain assessment and treatment recommendations, and false beliefs about biological differences between blacks and whites', *PNAS*, 113/16 (2016): 4296–301.

111   *and ethnic groups.* John A. Powell, '*Structural racism: building upon the insights of John Calmore*', *North Carolina Law Review*, 86 (*2008*): 791.

111   *a resounding success.* Norfolk, Suffolk and Cambridgeshire Strategic Health Authority, *Independent Inquiry into the Death of David Bennett* (Cambridge: Norfolk, Suffolk and Cambridgeshire Strategic Health Authority, 2003).

112   *one of them.* S. Wessely, *Modernising the Mental Health Act: Increasing Choice, Reducing Compulsion – Final Report of the Independent Review of the Mental Health Act 1983* (London: Department of Health and Social Care, *2018*), https://assets. publishing.service.gov.uk/government/uploads/system/ uploads/attachment_data/file/778897/Modernising_the_ Mental_Health_Act_-_increasing_choice__reducing_ compulsion.pdf.

118   *'sleep soundly'.* E. Fluckiger-Hawker, *Urnamma of Ur in Sumerian Literary Tradition* (Fribourg, Switzerland: University Press Fribourg, 1999).

118   *Ambroise Paré.* M. Ben-Ezra, 'Traumatic reactions from antiquity to the 16th century: was there a common denominator?', *Stress and Health*, 27 (2011): 223–40.

119   *British hospitals.* G. Weissman, 'The beast on my back', *London Review of Books*, 18/11 (1996).

120   *of the enemy.* S. Wessely, 'The life and death of Private Harry Farr', *Journal of the Royal Society of Medicine*, 99/9 (2006): 440–3.

120   *'disgrace to the soldier'. Report of the War Office Committee of Enquiry into 'Shell-Shock': Featuring a New Historical Essay on Shell Shock* (London [n. publ.]: 1922).

120   *'the US military'*. D. Summerfield, 'The invention of post-traumatic stress disorder and the social usefulness of a psychiatric category', *BMJ*, 322/7278 (2001): 95–8.

121   *'child abuse survivors'*. D. Fassin and R. Rechtman, *The Empire of Trauma: An Inquiry into the Condition of Victim-Hood* (Princeton, NJ: Princeton University Press, 2009).

121   *disability pension*. D. Summerfield, 'The invention of post-traumatic stress disorder'.

122   *'new definition'*. D. Fassin and R. Rechtman, *The Empire of Trauma*.

122   *'severe PTSD'*. De Jong K. et al., 'The trauma of war in Sierra Leone', *Lancet*, 355/9220 (2000): 2067–70.

126   *improved mental health*. S. Raghavan et al. 'Correlates of symptom reduction in treatment-seeking survivors of torture', *Psychological Trauma: Theory, Research, Practice, and Policy*, 5/4 (2013): 377–83.

128   *about the body*. Christopher C. Taylor, 'Ihahamuka: an indigenous medical condition among Rwandan genocide survivors', Oxford Handbooks Online (2015), https://www.oxfordhandbooks.com/view/10.1093/oxfordhb/9780199935420.001.0001/oxfordhb-9780199935420-e-51.

128   *Cambodian refugees*. D. E. Hinton and R. Lewis-Fernández, 'The cross-cultural validity of posttraumatic stress disorder: implications for DSM-5', *Depression and Anxiety*, 28/9 (2011): 783–801.

128   *fire welling up*. J. H. Jenkins and M. Valiente, 'Bodily transactions of the passions: *el calor* among Salvadoran women refugees', in T. J. Csordas, ed., *Embodiment and Experience: The Existential Ground of Culture and Self*

(Cambridge: CUP, 1994), pp. 163–82.

128   *'somatic symptoms'*. A. P. Levin, S. B. Kleinman and J. S. Adler, 'DSM-5 and posttraumatic stress disorder', *Journal of the American Academy of Psychiatry and the Law*, 42/2 (2014): 146–58.

129   *one recent academic paper*. I. R. Galatzer-Levy and R. A. Bryant, '636,120 ways to have posttraumatic stress disorder', *Perspectives on Psychological Science*, 8/6 (2013): 651–62.

131   *'coping methods'*. Angela Nickerson et al., 'Briefing paper: trauma and mental health in forcibly displaced populations', ISTSS (2017).

131   *'conventional treatment'*. Inter-Agency Standing Committee (IASC), *IASC Guidelines on Mental Health and Psychosocial Support in Emergency Settings* (Geneva: IASC, 2007).

131   *could potentially be harmful*. Harri Englund, 'Death, trauma and ritual: Mozambican refugees in Malawi', *Social Science & Medicine*, 46/9 (1998): 1165–74.

133   *'along those lines at all'*. D. Fassin and R. Rechtman, *The Empire of Trauma*.

138   *misconduct in public office*. Harmit Athwal and Jenny Bourne, eds, *Dying for Justice* (London: Institute of Race Relations, 2015).

139   *'a cardiac arrest'*. 'Mikey Powell inquest: Pathologist says "critical event" took place in police van', *Socialist Worker*, 1 Dec 2009.

139   *'It is not justice'*. Simon Basketter, 'Ten years on, police apologise over the death of Mikey Powell', *Socialist Worker*, 6 Sep 2013.

140   *deaths since 1996*. Charlie Mole, 'Unproven science used to "explain" deaths in police custody', Bureau of Investigative Journalism, 31 Jan 2012; Diane Taylor, 'Met police restraint contributed to death of mentally ill man, jury finds', *Guardian*,

9 Oct 2020; Richard Travers, 'Re: Terrence Arthur Albert Smith Deceased: Regulation 28 report to prevent future deaths', https://www.judiciary.uk/wp-content/uploads/2019/06/Terence-Smith-2019-0095_Redacted.pdf.

140 *800 cases a year*. Justin Jouvenal, '"Excited delirium" cited in dozens of deaths in police custody: is it real or a cover for brutality?', *Washington Post*, 6 May 2015.

140 *50 custodial deaths*. Michael Barajas, 'Is excited delirium syndrome a medical phenomenon, or a convenient cover for deaths in police custody?', *Texas Observer*, 16 Oct 2017.

140 *85 autopsy reports*. Alessandro Marazzi Sassoon, 'Excited delirium: rare and deadly syndrome or a condition to excuse deaths by police?', *Florida Today*, 24 Oct 2019.

141 *Journal of Forensic Sciences*. C. V. Wetli and D. A. Fishbain, 'Cocaine-induced psychosis and sudden death in recreational cocaine users', *Journal of Forensic Sciences*, 30/3 (1985): 873–80.

141 *'crack cocaine addicts'*. Barry Bearak, 'Eerie deaths of 17 women baffle Miami', *Los Angeles Times*, 14 May 1989.

142 *'adjacent to her neck'*. See https://www.muckrock.com/foi/miami-dade-county-7318/casefile-charles-henry-williams-medical-examiner-71458/#file-783416.

142 *'a thing like this'*. Barry Bearak, 'Eerie Deaths'.

143 *'another story'*. Gus Garcia-Roberts, 'Is excited delirium killing coked-up, stun-gunned Miamians?', *Miami New Times*, 15 Jul 2010.

143 *'pre-mortem state'*. ACEP Excited Delirium Task Force, *White Paper Report on Excited Delirium Syndrome* (Baltimore, MD: ACEP, 2009).

144 *'animal-like noises'*. Less-Lethal Devices Technology Working Group, *Special Panel Review of Excited Delirium*, National Institute of Justice (2011), www.justnet.org/pdf/exds-panel-report-final.pdf.

144 *'it's excited delirium'*. D. Costello, '"Excited delirium" as a cause of death', *Los Angeles Times*, 21 Apr 2003.

144 *Donald Lewis in 2005*. Supreme Court of the United States (ruling), Linda Lewis v. City of West Palm Beach, Florida et al., https://www.scotusblog.com/wp-content/uploads/2010/01/09-420_pet.pdf, 5 Oct 2009.

145 *'cocaine-induced excited delirium'*. United States District Court, Southern District of Florida, 'Order Denying Plaintiff's Motion for Summary Judgment', Case No. 06-81139-CIV-HURLEY/HOPKINS,https://www.govinfo.gov/content/pkg/USCOURTS-flsd-9_06-cv-81139/pdf/USCOURTS-flsd-9_06-cv-81139-0.pdf, 19 Mar 2008.

145 *over the past decade*. Elish Angiolini, *Report of the Independent Review of Deaths and Serious Incidents in Police Custody*, Home Office (2017).

146 *a civilised society*. INQUEST, 'Inquest into the death of Terry Smith concludes neglect contributed to death involving excessive restraint by Surrey Police', 5 Jul 2018, https://www.inquest.org.uk/terry-smith-conclusion.

146 *'level of adrenaline'*. Richard Travers, 'Regulation 28 report'.

146 *10% of police custody deaths*. Angiolini, *Report of the Independent Review*.

146 *'contribute to the deaths'*. IOPC, *Deaths During or Following Police Contact: Statistics for England and Wales 2020/21* (London: IOPC, 2021).

147 *continue to occur*. Angiolini, *Report of the Independent Review*.

147 *deaths in custody*. INQUEST, 'BAME deaths in police custody', https://www.inquest.org.uk/bame-deaths-in-police-custody.

147 *'was unsuitable'*. Vikram Dodd, 'Sean Rigg death in custody: police used unnecessary force, jury finds', *Guardian*, 1 Aug 2012.

147   *8 minutes and 15 seconds.* See '8 minutes, 46 seconds became a
      symbol in George Floyd's death; the exact time is less clear',
      The New York Times, 18 Jun 2020.

147   *'delirium or whatever'.* Richard A. Oppel Jr. and Lazaro Gamio,
      'Minneapolis police use force against black people at 7 times
      the rate of whites', *The New York Times*, 3 Jun 2020.

147   *involve black men.* Laura Sullivan, 'Death by excited delirium:
      diagnosis or coverup?', NPR, 26 Feb 2007, https://www.
      npr.org/templates/story/story.php?storyId=7608386&t=
      1591173997062&t=1633356907396.

148   *in his apartment.* The quotations from here to the end of this
      section are all from *Braidwood Commission on the Death of
      Robert Dziekanski*, 2010, https://opcc.bc.ca/wp-content/
      uploads/2017/04/Why-The-Robert-Dziekanski-Tragedy.
      pdf.

152   *could have been used.* 'How Safe Are Taser Weapons?', Axon,
      https://global.axon.com/how-safe-are-taser-weapons.

152   *alternative to firearms.* Amnesty International, *"Less Than
      Lethal"? The Use of Stun Weapons in US Law Enforcement*
      (London: Amnesty International, 2008).

153   *followed taser use.* J. Szep, T. Reid and P. Eisler, 'How Taser
      inserts itself into investigations involving its weapons', *Reuters*,
      24   Aug   2017,   https://www.reuters.com/investigates/
      special-report/usa-taser-experts.

153   *'physical struggle'.* 'Taser Handheld CEW warnings,
      instructions, and information: law enforcement',
      Axon, 30 Oct 2018, p. 2, https://axon.cdn.prismic.io/
      axon%2F3cd3d65a-7500-4667-a9a8-0549fc3226c7_law-
      enforcement-warnings%2B8-5x11.pdf.

153   *'see these signs'.* Laura Sullivan, 'Tasers implicated in excited
      delirium deaths,' NPR, 27 Feb 2007, https://www.npr.
      org/templates/story/story.php?storyId=7622314?storyId=7

622314&t=1581943362734&t=1626191593953.

153   *'according to a lawsuit'*. M. B. Pell, 'Across the U.S., high-profile deaths lead to stun-gun case settlements', *Reuters*, 24 Aug 2017, https://www.reuters.com/article/us-usa-taser-cases/across-the-u-s-high-profile-deaths-lead-to-stun-gun-case-settlements-idUSKCN1B4188.

154   *future decisions.* W. R. Oliver, 'The effect of threat of litigation on forensic pathologist diagnostic decision making', *American Journal of Forensic Medicine and Pathology*, 32/4 (2011): 383–6.

154   *'consistent with excited delirium syndrome'*. Amnesty International, *"Less than Lethal?"*

154   *'this type of litigation'*. Tim Reid and Paula Seligson, 'Taser's defense tactics include lawsuits against coroners and experts', *Reuters*, 24 Aug 2017, https://www.reuters.com/article/us-usa-taser-strikeback-idUSKCN1B4182

155   *'state of Colorado'*. 'Our Misson', Police1, https://www.police1.com/info/about.

155   *'when feasible'*. Mark Kroll, Jeffrey Ho, and Gary Vilke, '8 Facts about excited delirium syndrome (ExDS)', Police1, Mar 2019 https://www.police1.com/police-training/articles/8-facts-about-excited-delirium-syndrome-exds-nutDY9i2C1ATmeV5/.

155   *'lives can be saved'*. J. Szep et al., 'How Taser inserts itself'.

155   *'12-month stretch'*. Bernice Yeung, 'Taser's delirium defense: how lawyers used junk science to explain away stun-gun deaths', Mother Jones, Mar/Apr 2009, https://www.motherjones.com/politics/2009/02/tasers-delirium-defense.

155   *'earned $267,000'*. J. Szep et al., 'How Taser inserts itself'.

155   *'worth over $3 million'*. See https://gb.wallmine.com/people/3026/mark-w-kroll/.

156   *drawn or aimed.* Home Office, 'Police use of force statistics,

England and Wales: April 2019 to March 2020', *Home Office Statistical Bulletin*, 37/20.

156 *8,000 CEDs*. Mattha Busby, 'Rights groups quit police body over stun gun use against BAME people', *Guardian*, 17 Apr 2020.

156 *will carry CEDs by 2022*. Vikram Dodd, 'Met police officer investigated after man shot with Taser stun gun is left paralysed', *Guardian*, 15 May 2020.

156 *in the Metropolitan police force area*. Home Office, 'Police use of force statistics'.

156 *every criminal case*. D. E. Shelton, Y. S. Kim and G. Barak. 'A study of juror expectations and demands concerning scientific evidence: does the "*CSI* Effect" exist?', *Vanderbilt Journal of Entertainment and Technology Law*, 9/2 (2006): 331–68.

157 *intoxication or trauma*. D. C. Mash et al., 'Brain biomarkers for identifying excited delirium as a cause of sudden death', *Forensic Science International*, 190/1–3 (2009): e13–9.

157 *'trip the switch*. Aria Pearson, 'Can excited delirium get cops off the hook?', *New Scientist*, 5 Aug 2009.

157 *refused to disclose her earnings*. Gus Garcia-Roberts, 'Is excited delirium killing coked-up, stun-gunned Miamians?'.

157 *calls him a 'mentor'*. J. Szep et al., 'How Taser inserts itself'.

158 *so-called excited delirium*. M. M. Johnson et al., 'Increased heat shock protein 70 gene expression in the brains of cocaine-related fatalities may be reflective of postdrug survival and intervention rather than excited delirium', *Journal of Forensic Sciences*, 57/6 (2012): 1519–23.

158 *must be collected ASAP*. J. Szep et al., 'How Taser inserts itself'.

159 *Nobody was charged*. Ibid.

160 *'into the road'*. Shiv Malik, 'Police ignored pleas for ambulance, say family of man who died in custody', *Guardian*, 30 Sep 2011.

160   *'young black man'*. 'Inquest into death of Jacob Michael in police custody in Runcorn to begin Monday 1st October', 27 Sep 2012, https://www.inquest.org.uk/jacob-michael-inquest-opens.

160   *died of excited delirium*. Shiv Malik, '"Excited delirium" finding in custody death angers parents', *Guardian*, 1 Feb 2012.

160   *'rang the police for help'*. Malik, '"Excited delirium" finding'.

161   *'hit him with batons'*. Malik, 'Police ignored pleas'.

161   *serious mental illness*. Independent Advisory Panel on Deaths in Custody, *The Royal College of Emergency Medicine Best Practice Guideline: Guidelines for the Management of Excited Delirium / Acute Behavioural Disturbance (ABD)* (London: RCEM, 2016).

165   *Section 136 detainments*. B. Reveruzzi and S. Pilling, *Street Triage: Report on the Evaluation of Nine Pilot Schemes in England* (London: UCL Press, 2016).

165   *West Midlands Police area*. Ibid.

172   *shred of doubt*. 'WHO releases new International Classification of Diseases (ICD 11)', WHO, 'News', 18 Jun 2018, https://www.who.int/news/item/18-06-2018-who-releases-new-international-classification-of-diseases-(icd-11).

172   *'how to treat it'*. Jessica Pupillo, 'PANDAS/PANS treatments, awareness evolve, but some experts skeptical', *AAP News*, 28 Mar 2017, https://www.aappublications.org/news/2017/03/28/Pandas032817.

172   *'believer' in the condition*. Rachel Zamzow, 'Infected mind: a rare autoimmune condition spurs controversy, forges new frontiers, *Unearthed*, 7 May 2015.

172   *'20 years of controversy'*. Jessica Pupillo, 'PANDAS/PANS treatments'.

173   *posted on Facebook*. Brendan Borrell, 'How a controversial

condition called PANDAS is gaining ground on autism', *Spectrum News*, 8 Jan 2020.

173 *the Joint Commission.* See https://www.facebook.com/ login/?next=https%3A%2F%2Fwww.facebook.com%2F pandasnetwork%2Fposts%2Fcollectively-we-have-heard- and-share-the-frustration-around-the-recent-grand- rou%2F1863321510381765%2F.

173 *'I chose not to'.* Brendan Borrell, 'Controversial condition called PANDAS'.

174 *until sometime later.* K. J. Rothman and S. Greenland, 'Causation and causal inference in epidemiology', *American Journal of Public Health*, 95/supplement 1 (2005): S144–S150.

176 *the mitral region.* J. Schwartzman, J. B. Zaontz and H. Lubow, 'Chorea minor: preliminary report on six patients treated with combined ACTH and cortisone', *Journal of Pediatrics*, 43/3 (1953): 278–89.

178 *has never been established.* H. S. Singer, 'Autoantibody-associated movement disorders in children: proven and proposed', *Seminars in Pediatric Neurology*, 24/3 (2017): 168–79.

178 *streptococcal infection.* S. E. Swedo et al., 'High prevalence of obsessive-compulsive symptoms in patients with Sydenham's chorea', *American Journal of Psychiatry*, 146/2 (1989): 246–9.

178 *in February 1998.* S. E. Swedo et al., 'Pediatric autoimmune neuropsychiatric disorders associated with streptococcal infections: clinical description of the first 50 cases', *American Journal of Psychiatry*, 155/2 (1998): 264–71. (Published correction in 155(4): 578.)

179 *half of children.* D. R. Johnson et al., 'The human immune response to streptococcal extracellular antigens: clinical, diagnostic, and potential pathogenetic implications', *Clinical Infectious Diseases*, 50/4 (2010): 481–90.

179 *(up to 20% of children).* On OCD, see G. Krebs and I.

Heyman, 'Obsessive-compulsive disorder in children and adolescents', *Archives of Disease in Childhood*, 100 (2015): 495–9; on tic disorders, see L. Scahill, M. Specht and C. Page, 'The prevalence of tic disorders and clinical characteristics in children', *JOCRD*, 3/4 (2014): 394–400.

179   *obsessive-compulsive symptoms.* L. K. Mell, R. L. Davis and D. Owens, 'Association between streptococcal infection and obsessive-compulsive disorder, Tourette's syndrome, and tic disorder', *Pediatrics*, 116/1 (2005): 56–60.

179   *autoimmune process.* H. S. Singer et al., 'Tourette syndrome study group: serial immune markers do not correlate with clinical exacerbations in pediatric autoimmune neuropsychiatric disorders associated with streptococcal infections', *Pediatrics*, 121/6 (2008): 1198–205.

180   *metabolic triggers.* O. Köhler-Forsberg et al., 'A nationwide study in Denmark of the association between treated infections and the subsequent risk of treated mental disorders in children and adolescents', *JAMA Psychiatry*, 76/3 (2019): 271–9.

181   *weeks and months.* Chico Harlan, 'Mom fights for answers on what's wrong with her son', *Pittsburgh Post-Gazette*, 23 Jul 2006.

181   *'Coughs and Convulsions'.* C. E. Kellett, 'Sir Thomas Browne and the disease called the Morgellons', *Annals of Medical History*, 7/5 (1935): 467–79.

182   *'living at home'.* 'Living with Morgellons', Morgellons Research Foundation, 30 Apr 2014, https://www.morgellons.org/life_with/.

183   *'over the internet'.* R. Bartholomew and P. Hassall, *A Colorful History of Popular Delusions* (Amherst, NY: Prometheus, 2015).

183   *'exploring this problem'.* Chico Harlan, 'Mom fights for answers'.

184   *in bed for a year.* Matt Diehl, 'It's a Joni Mitchell concert, sans Joni', *Los Angeles Times*, 22 Apr 2010.

184   *'study the condition'.* Will Storr, 'Morgellons: A hidden epidemic or mass hysteria?', *Guardian*, 7 May 2011.

184   *research the condition in earnest.* B. Fair, 'Morgellons: contested illness, diagnostic compromise and medicalisation', *Sociology of Health & Illness*, 32 (2010): 597–612.

184   *in their database.* See https://www.morgellons.org.

185   *'delusional infestation'.* M. L. Pearson et al., 'Clinical, epidemiologic, histopathologic and molecular features of an unexplained dermopathy', PLOS ONE, 7/1 (2012): e29908.

191   *'medicalization of misery'.* See G. E. Ehrlich, 'Pain is real; fibromyalgia isn't', *Journal of Rheumatology*, 30/8 (2003): 1666–7; and N. M. Hadler, '"Fibromyalgia" and the medicalization of misery', ibid.: 1668–70.

191   *1980s and after.* F. Wolfe and B. Walitt, 'Culture, science and the changing nature of fibromyalgia', *Nature Reviews Rheumatology*, 9/12 (2013): 751–5.

191   *a physician's examination.* F. Wolfe et al., 'The American College of Rheumatology 1990 criteria for the classification of fibromyalgia: report of the multicenter criteria committee', *Arthritis & Rheumatology*, 33/2 (1990): 160–72.

191   *one rheumatologist.* J. L. Quintner and M. L. Cohen, 'Fibromyalgia falls foul of a fallacy', *Lancet*, 353/9158 (1999): 1092–4.

192   *'the wrong thing'.* Alex Berenson, 'Drug approved. Is disease real?', *The New York Times*, 14 Jan 2008.

192   *'a substantial or clinically meaningful way'.* F. Wolfe and B. Walitt, 'Culture, science'.

192   *prescribed painkillers.* K. E. Mansfield et al., 'A systematic review and meta-analysis of the prevalence of chronic widespread pain in the general population', *Pain*, 157/1 (2016): 55–64.

192   *credibility of the diagnosis.* See G. T. Jones et al., 'The prevalence
of fibromyalgia in the general population: a comparison
of the American College of Rheumatology 1990, 2010,
and modified 2010 classification criteria', *Arthritis &
Rheumatology*, 67/2 (2015): 568–75; and F. Wolfe et al., 'The
prevalence and characteristics of fibromyalgia in the general
population', ibid., 38/1 (1995): 19–28.

192   *new drug market.* K. K. Barker, 'Listening to Lyrica: contested
illnesses and pharmaceutical determinism', *Social Science &
Medicine*, 73/6 (2011): 833–42.

193   *'became real to people'.* Alex Berenson, 'Drug Approved'.

193   *their own families.* K. K. Barker, 'Listening to Lyrica'.

193   *approved for fibromyalgia. Pfizer Inc. 2007 Financial Report* and
Pfizer Inc. 2009 Financial Report, see https://investors.pfizer.
com/financials/annual-reports/.

194   *an eleven-fold increase.* Sarah Marsh, 'Pregabalin, known
as "new valium", to be made class C drug after deaths',
Guardian, 21 Sep 2017.

194   *'visit your GP'.* See https://www.nhs.uk/conditions/
fibromyalgia.

194   *for most people.* S. Derry et al., 'Pregabalin for pain in
fibromyalgia in adults', *Cochrane Database of Systematic
Reviews*, 9 (2016), article no. CD011790.

195   *'a warm glow'.* K. K. Barker, 'Listening to Lyrica'.

195   *41% rise in fatalities.* ONS, 'Deaths related to drug poisoning
in England and Wales: 2020 registrations', https://
www.ons.gov.uk/peoplepopulationandcommunity/
birthsdeathsandmarriages/deaths/bulletins/
deathsrelatedtodrugpoisoninginenglandandwales/2020.

195   *'my fibromyalgia isn't real'.* See https://themighty.
com/2015/11/a-letter-to-someone-who-thinks-
fibromyalgia-isnt-real/.

196 *'four drugs'*. US Department of Justice, 'Justice department announces largest health care fraud settlement in its history', 2 Sep 2009, https://www.justice.gov/opa/pr/justice-department-announces-largest-health-care-fraud-settlement-its-history.

196 *'three weeks of Pfizer's sales'*. Gardiner Harris, 'Pfizer pays $2.3 billion to settle marketing case', *The New York Times*, 2 Sep 2009.

197 *have been inconsistent*. H. S. Singer et al., 'Tourette syndrome study group'.

197 *'a pastry chef'*. Pamela Weintraub, 'Understanding PANS, a frightening condition that can turn children inexplicably violent', *Discover*, 3 Jan 2019.

197 *superior to a placebo*. K. A. Williams et al., 'Randomized, controlled trial of intravenous immunoglobulin for pediatric autoimmune neuropsychiatric disorders associated with streptococcal infections', *Journal of the American Academy of Child and Adolescent Psychiatry*, 55/10 (2016): 860–7.e2.

197 *perceived benefit*. S. Sigra, E. Hesselmark and S. Bejerot, 'Treatment of PANDAS and PANS: a systematic review', *Neuroscience & Biobehavioral Reviews*, 86 (2018): 51–65.

198 *gut damage*. D. L. Gilbert, J. W. Mink and H. S. Singer, 'A pediatric neurology perspective on pediatric autoimmune neuropsychiatric disorder associated with streptococcal infection and pediatric acute-onset neuropsychiatric syndrome', *Journal of Pediatrics*, 199 (2018): 243–51.

198 *adverse effects*. J. Kubota et al., 'Predictive factors of first dosage intravenous immunoglobulin-related adverse effects in children', PLOS ONE, 15/1 (2020): e0227796.

198 *strokes and meningitis*. J. S. Orange et al., 'Use of intravenous immunoglobulin in human disease: a review of evidence by members of the Primary Immunodeficiency Committee of

the American Academy of Allergy, Asthma and Immunology',
Journal of Allergy and Clinical Immunology, 117 (2006): 525–53.

198 *OCD and tic disorders.* See for instance Adam Finn, Nigel
Curtis and Andrew J. Pollard, eds, *Hot Topics in Infection and
Immunity in Children V* (New York: Springer Media, 2008),
p. 205.

199 *children are affected.* Jessica Pupillo, 'PANDAS/PANS
treatments'.

199 *'kindergarten class'.* Kira Peikoff, 'My son almost lost his mind
from strep throat', *Cosmopolitan*, 1 Oct 2014, https://www.
cosmopolitan.com/lifestyle/news/a31681/my-son-lost-
his-mind-from-strep-throat/.

199 *'have drugs for that'.* R. Volansky and S. T. Shulman, 'PANDAS
to CANS: evolution of a controversial disorder', *Infectious
Diseases in Children*, 25/10 (2012): 1.

199 *'not necessarily correct'.* R. Zanzow, 'Infected mind: a rare
autoimmune condition spurs controversy, forges new
frontiers', *Unearthed*, 7 May 2015, https://unearthedmag.
wordpress.com/2015/05/07/infected-mind-a-rare-
autoimmune-condition-spurs-controversy-forges-new-
frontiers/.

203 *1.3% of women.* K. B. Kuchenbaecker et al., 'Risks of breast,
ovarian, and contralateral breast cancer for *BRCA1* and
BRCA2 mutation carriers', *JAMA,* 317/23 (2017): 2402–
16.

204 *mother or sister.* T. J. Padamsee et al., 'Decision making for
breast cancer prevention among women at elevated risk',
Breast Cancer Research, 19/1 (2017): 34.

208 *they have a VUS.* C. G. Selkirk et al., 'Cancer genetic testing
panels for inherited cancer susceptibility: the clinical
experience of a large adult genetics practice', *Familial Cancer*,
13 (2014): 527–36.

208   *the same news.* T. D. Pottinger et al., 'Pathogenic and uncertain genetic variants have clinical cardiac correlates in diverse biobank participants', *Journal of the American Heart Association*, 9/3 (2020): e013808.

208   *from white people.* Lily Hoffman-Andrews, 'The known unknown: the challenges of genetic variants of uncertain significance in clinical practice', *Journal of Law and the Biosciences*, 4/3 (2017): 648–57.

208   *considered a VUS.* D. M. Eccles et al., 'ENIGMA clinical working group: BRCA1 and BRCA2 genetic testing-pitfalls and recommendations for managing variants of uncertain clinical significance', *Annals of Oncology*, 26/10 (2015): 2057–65.

208   *$6.36 billion by 2028.* BIS Research, *Global Direct-to-Consumer Genetic Testing (DTC-GT) Market: Focus on Direct-to-Consumer Genetic Testing Market by Product Type, Distribution Channel, 15 Countries Mapping and Competitive Landscape – Analysis and Forecast, 2019–2028*, 2019.

209   *routine clinical care.* See Department for Business, Energy & Industrial Strategy and Department for Health & Social Care, 'Genome UK: the future of healthcare', 26 Sep 2020, https://www.gov.uk/government/publications/genome-uk-the-future-of-healthcare/genome-uk-the-future-of-healthcare.

209   *BRCA mutation.* A. W. Kurian et al., 'Gaps in incorporating germline genetic testing into treatment decision-making for early-stage breast cancer', *Journal of Clinical Oncology*, 35/20 (2017): 2232–9.

210   *'black or white'.* J. Vos et al., 'The counsellees' view of an unclassified variant in BRCA1/2: recall, interpretation, and impact on life', *Psycho-oncology*, 17/8 (2008): 822–30.

210   *classification system.* D. M. Eccles et al., 'ENIGMA clinical working group'.

211   *'in such women'*. K. L. Jones et al., 'Outcome in offspring of chronic alcoholic women', *Lancet*, 1/7866 (1974): 1076–8.

213   *'liquor a day'*. E. L. Abel, 'Fetal alcohol syndrome: a cautionary note', *Current Pharmaceutical Design*, 12/12 (2006): 1521–9.

214   *when you are pregnant*. Department of Health & Social Care, 'New alcohol guidelines show increased risk of cancer', 'News', 8 Jan 2016, https://www.gov.uk/government/news/new-alcohol-guidelines-show-increased-risk-of-cancer.

214   *'childbearing age'*. WHO, 'Global alcohol action plan 2022–30 to strengthen implementation of the global strategy to reduce the harmful use of alcohol, first draft, Jun 2021' (WHO, 2021), p. 17.

214   *Between 40% and 80% of women*. L. M. O'Keeffe et al., 'Prevalence and predictors of alcohol use during pregnancy: findings from international multicentre cohort studies', *BMJ Open*, 5/7 (2015): e006323.

216   *all in one go*. L. Mamluk et al., 'Low alcohol consumption and pregnancy and childhood outcomes: time to change guidelines indicating apparently "safe" levels of alcohol during pregnancy? A systematic review and meta-analyses', *BMJ Open*, 7/7 (2017): e015410.

217   *'precautionary approach'*. Science Media Centre, 'Expert reaction to study looking at potential harms of light drinking in pregnancy', 11 Sep 2017, https://www.sciencemediacentre.org/expert-reaction-to-study-looking-at-potential-harms-of-light-drinking-in-pregnancy/.

217   *in West Germany*. Marco Martuzzi and Joel A. Tickner, eds, *The Precautionary Principle: Protecting Public Health, the Environment and the Future of our Children* (WHO, 2004).

217   *'environmental degradation'*. UN, *Report of the United Nations Conference on Environment and Development*, 12 Aug 1992.

218   *greater prominence.* Royal Society for Public Health, *Labelling the Point: Towards Better Alcohol Health Information* (London: RSPH, 2018).

219   *'threat to our survival'*. Edward Adam Strecker, *Their Mothers' Sons: The Psychiatrist Examines an American Problem* (New York, 1946), p. 219.

219   *probability and outcomes.* A. Leppo, D. Hecksher and K. Tryggvesson, '"Why take chances?" Advice on alcohol intake to pregnant and non-pregnant women in four Nordic countries', *Health, Risk & Society*, 16/6 (2014): 512–29.

220   *mice offspring.* R. T. Bottom, C. W. Abbott and K. J. Huffman, 'Rescue of ethanol-induced FASD-like phenotypes via prenatal co-administration of choline', *Neuropharmacology*, 168 (2020): 107990.

220   *consumption before pregnancy.* L. Zuccolo et al., 'Preconception and prenatal alcohol exposure from mothers and fathers drinking and head circumference: results from the Norwegian Mother-Child Study (MoBa)' *Scientific Reports*, 7 (2016): 39535.

220   *'high-risk occupations'*. BMA, *Alcohol and Pregnancy: Preventing and Managing Fetal Alcohol Spectrum Disorders* (London: BMA, 2016).

221   *'that is prevented'*. D. Wilkinson et al., 'Protecting future children from in-utero harm', *Bioethics*, 30 (2016): 425–32.

221   *'habitual or excessive'*. N. K. Seiler, 'Alcohol and pregnancy: CDC's health advice and the legal rights of pregnant women', *Public health reports*, 131/4 (2016): 623–7.

221   *more babies are born prematurely.* M. S. Subbaraman and S. C. M. Roberts, 'Costs associated with policies regarding alcohol use during pregnancy: results from 1972–2015 vital statistics', *PLOS ONE*, 14/5 (2019): e0215670.

222   *alcohol or drug use.* S. C. Roberts and A. Nuru-Jeter, 'Universal

screening for alcohol and drug use and racial disparities in child protective services reporting', *Journal of Behavioral Health Services & Research*, 39/1 (2012): 3–16.

222   *reunited with them.* K. L. H. Harp and A. M. Bunting, 'The racialized nature of child welfare policies and the social control of black bodies', *Social Politics*, 27/2 (2020): 258–81.

223   *'public health message'.* BMA, *Alcohol and pregnancy.*

223   *'not grow properly'.* Lorna Marsh, 'Alcohol during pregnancy', BabyCentre UK, Apr 2021, https://www.babycentre.co.uk/ a3542/alcohol–during–pregnancy.

223   *you're pregnant.* Drinkaware, 'Alcohol and pregnancy', https:// www.drinkaware.co.uk/facts/health-effects-of-alcohol/ alcohol-fertility-and-pregnancy/alcohol-and-pregnancy.

223   *'no, not really'.* NCT, 'Alcohol: can I drink when I'm pregnant?', https://www.nct.org.uk/pregnancy/food-and-nutrition/alcohol-can-i-drink-when-im-pregnant.

224   *'future health'.* NHS Start 4 Life, 'Can I drink alcohol during pregnancy?', https://www.nhs.uk/start4life/pregna ncy/alcohol/.

224   *'with their children'.* NOFAS, 'Alcohol and pregnancy advice in new book is flawed and harmful', Cision PR Newswire, https://www.prnewswire.com/news-releases/alcohol-and-pregnancy-advice-in-new-book-is-flawed-and-harmful-220563061.html.

225   *book's publisher.* See https://www.facebook.com/nofas/ posts/emily-oster-posted-an-article-today-attacking-nofas-and-people-with-fasd-who-hav/552676901452320/.

225   *run-ins with the law.* T. W. Tsang and E. J. Elliott, 'High global prevalence of alcohol use during pregnancy and fetal alcohol syndrome indicates need for urgent action', *Lancet Global Health*, 5/3 (2017): e232-e233.

232   *passionately upheld.* Patrick Strudwick, 'Psychiatrists have

issued a historic admission of the harm done by aversion therapy', BuzzFeed, 16 Oct 2017, https://www.buzzfeed. com/patrickstrudwick/uk-psychiatrists-have-issued-an- historic-admission-of-the.

Acknowledgements

A special thank you to Will Francis, my extraordinary literary agent. I feel so lucky to be able to regularly draw on your superb intellectual wisdom. Yet again, the agent of all agents. The terrific team at Janklow & Nesbit champion their authors with care and kindness – thank you to Ren Balcombe, Mairi Friesen-Escandell, Maimy Suleiman, Ellis Hazelgrove, Michael Steger and Kirsty Gordon.

To the editors at Granta – I'm grateful to Anne Meadows for placing her faith in *The Imaginary Patient* and helping to consolidate its ideas; to Rowan Cope for her incisive commentary and wonderfully insightful critique; and to Jason Arthur who has seen this book through to completion. Thanks, too, to the rest of the Granta team who work behind the scenes to set the stage for every book they publish.

Jonathan Metzl generously took the time to meet with me during a visit to London. His book *Protest Psychosis* informed so much of my writing on racialised diagnoses both in the US and closer to home. I'm indebted to Suman Fernando, a psychiatrist who has spent decades highlighting the devastating labelling of black men with a diagnosis of cannabis psychosis. My investigation into that diagnosis led me to the gifted photographer and journalist Derek Bishton, one of the team who created the groundbreaking 1978 project *Handsworth Self Portrait*. Derek walked the streets of Handsworth with me, introduced me to Hector Pinkney, and together their vivid stories brought the tumultuous events of Autumn 1985 into sharp focus.

Sarah Carr provided an illuminating personal perspective for this book, and a professional one too. Her research with Helen Spandler explores the experiences of psychiatric survivors who identify as LGBTQ+. The hidden histories unveiled by Sarah and Helen exhibit archival activism at its best.

I am indebted to the talented journalists at Reuters who put together the 'Shock Tactics' series. They have done brave, arduous and diligent investigative work. Their eighteen-month examination of fatalities reviewed thousands of court records, and analysed hundreds of autopsies and wrongful death lawsuits filed against police. It ultimately uncovered the stories behind deaths and litigations linked to stun guns. Those journalists are Jason Szep, Peter Eisler, Tim Reid, Lisa Girion, Grant Smith, Linda So, M. B. Pell and Charles Levinson. Without their work, we never would have known.

I thank the Médecins Sans Frontières team at Moria who, in enormously challenging times, enabled me to meet Ayesha and her family, and the others on the island whose stories you have read here. Closer to home, Jennifer Cimerman at the Marie Keating Foundation helped out when I started delving into the impact of BRCA diagnoses. The foundation's advice line and support groups in Ireland have proven to be utterly transformative for people with cancer and their families.

Paul Allchin, reference specialist at the British Library set me up strongly for the research journey that lay ahead. SciHub did what SciHub should do. The Society of Authors provided much-needed backing at a vital time. Gesche Ipsen examined the manuscript for this book with the meticulous attention and judicious eagle-eye one hopes for from a copy-editor.

Declan Barry was instrumental in first discussing and deliberating the ideas that eventually made it into this book. A note of gratitude to the many other friends who have helped along the way, especially Jen Spillane, Jo Randall, Patrick Page, Sharon Murray, Davina Sharma and Sarah Myers.

Thank you to my family for their enduring and unconditional support of my work, even though that work has sometimes been a little riskier than they would have liked.

And finally, thank you to Matt for, well, come to think of it, absolutely everything.

Index